Other Books by
Sharman Apt Russell

An Obsession with Butterflies

Anatomy of a Rose

Songs of the Fluteplayer

Kill the Cowboy

When the Land Was Young

SCHAUMBURG TOWNSHIP DISTRICT LIBRARY

W9-CCO-183

WITHDRAWN

Schaumburg Township District Library
130 South Roselle Road
Schaumburg, Illinois 60193

HUNGER

HUNGER

An Unnatural History

SHARMAN APT RUSSELL

BASIC
BOOKS

A Member of the Perseus Books Group
New York

SCHAUMBURG TOWNSHIP DISTRICT LIBRARY
130 SOUTH ROSELLE ROAD
SCHAUMBURG, ILLINOIS 60193

363.809
Russel, S

3 1257 01604 9537

Copyright © 2005 by Sharman Apt Russell
Published by Basic Books
A Member of the Perseus Books Group

All rights reserved. Printed in the United States of America. No part of this
book may be reproduced in any manner whatsoever without written
permission except in the case of brief quotations embodied in critical
articles and reviews. For information, address Basic Books, 387 Park Avenue
South, New York, NY 10016-8810.

Books published by Basic Books are available at special discounts for bulk
purchases in the United States by corporations, institutions, and other
organizations. For more information, please contact the Special Markets
Department at the Perseus Books Group, 11 Cambridge Center, Cambridge
MA 02142, or call (617) 252-5298 or (800) 255-1514, or e-mail
special.markets@perseusbooks.com.

Designed by Brent Wilcox
Text set in 11.25-point Fairfield Light

Library of Congress Cataloging-in-Publication Data
Russell, Sharman Apt.
    Hunger : an unnatural history / Sharman Apt Russell.
        p.   cm.
    Includes bibliographical references.
    ISBN-13 978-0-465-07163-0
    ISBN-10 0-465-07163-5 (hardcover : alk. paper)
    1. Hunger—Social aspects.   2. Fasting—Social aspects.
    3. Weight loss—Social aspects.   I. Title.
    HN8.R88   2005
    363.8'09—dc22

                                                  2005008034

            05 06 07 / 10 9 8 7 6 5 4 3 2 1

To my family

CONTENTS

THE
HUNGER ARTISTS

HUNGER IS A COUNTRY WE ENTER EVERY DAY, like a commuter across a friendly border. We wake up hungry We endure that for a matter of minutes before we break our fast. Later we may skip lunch and miss dinner. We may not eat for religious reasons. We may not eat before surgery. We may go on a three-day fast to cleanse ourselves of toxins and boredom. We may go on a longer fast to imitate Christ in the desert or to lose weight. We may go on a hunger strike. If we are lost at sea, if we have lost our job, if we are at war, we may not be hungry by choice.

Our body is a circle of messages: communication, feedback, updates. Hunger and satiety are the most basic of these. Every day, we learn more about how this system works. We know what hormones run through the blood screaming, "Eat!" We know which ones follow murmuring, "Enough." We know that it is relatively easy to repress the signal for enough. A gene malfunctions, and a three-year-old girl weighs a hundred pounds: her body does not tell her when to stop eating. That signal is complexly influenced by genetics, chemistry, and culture. For many of us, it has become blurred. Our body doesn't give us the news or doesn't give it with enough emphasis.

The signal for hunger is much, much harder to turn off. We are omnivores with an oversized brain that requires a lot of energy. We are not specialized in how we get our food. Instead, we are always willing, always alert, always ready with a rock or digging stick. We are happy to snack all day long. We are particularly drawn to the high-caloric bit of fat around the deer's kidney and the sweet taste of berries. Our love of fat and sugar has been associated with the same chemical responses that underlie our addictions to alcohol and drugs; this cycle of addiction may have developed to encourage eating behavior. We hunger easily, we find food, we get a chemical reward. Then we're hungry again. That's good, because the next time we look for food, we may not find it. Better keep eating while you can.

Human beings evolved for a bad day of hunting, a bad week of hunting, a bad crop, a bad year of crops. We were hungry even in that first Garden of Eden, what some anthropologists call the "Paleoterrific," a world full of large animals and relatively few people. Paleolithic bones and teeth occasionally show an unnatural pause in growth, a sign of food shortage. Our diet didn't get better as our population grew and the big-game species died out. In the Mesolithic, we foraged more intensively for plants and hunted smaller game with new tools like nets and snares. In the Neolithic, we invented agriculture, which sparked the rise of cities. There is no evidence that any of these changes reduced the odds of starvation or malnutrition. A more common trend seems to be that small-game hunters were shorter and less nourished than their Paleolithic ancestors, farmers less healthy than hunters-and-gatherers, and city-dwellers less robust than farmers. We just kept getting hungrier.

It's no wonder we are programmed to pound the table and demand dinner. The exceptions to this are usually extreme: infection, disease, terminal illness. For most of us, at regular times, the body shouts, "Feed me, damn it!" Deprived, the body sulks. The body exacts its petty revenge. Finally, with extraordinary cunning, and with something that approaches grace, the body turns to the business of the day, beginning what scientists call "the metabolic gymnastics" by which it can survive without food.

If you are healthy and well-nourished, you can live this way for sixty days. You can live much longer if you have more fat to break down. The rhythms of your life will change: your heartbeat, your hormones, your thoughts. Your brain will switch to a new energy source, something rare and wonderful, something only humans do and a few lactating ungulates. You will start consuming yourself, but precisely, carefully, with such orchestration.

You are built to be hungry and you are built to withstand hunger. You know exactly what to do.

. . .

In his short story "A Hunger Artist," written in 1922, Franz Kafka described a professional faster in the late nineteenth century who lived publicly in a small cage, eating nothing for days and then weeks. His performance ended with a grand finale on the fortieth day when "the flower-bedecked cage was opened" and an adoring audience waited as a military band played and doctors examined the emaciated patient. The results of their study were announced through a megaphone. Finally, two blissful and giddy young ladies appeared to escort the hunger artist to a carefully chosen meal.

In Kafka's story, the faster does not want to stop fasting. He is in fine form. There are no limits to his capacity! His manager insists, and the hunger artist has no choice but to eat, recover, and begin the show again in a new town with a new audience. The model for this character may have been the flamboyant Giovanni Succi, who fasted professionally over thirty times in all the major capitals of Europe. Succi believed himself possessed by a benign spirit, which enabled him to live without food. Between shows, he was quietly and regularly admitted into the insane asylum. On December 21, 1890, in New York, the *Daily Tribune* described how he broke a forty-five-day fast:

> Scores of men and women stood in the room waiting to say or do something or see something done at the moment when the fast should end. Expectations were on tip toe. . . . At 8-o'clock sharp, Succi arose from his couch and then it seemed as if the persons looking at him were welcoming back from the grave a long-lost brother. Cheer followed cheer and hands vied with feet in making noise. Succi, his hands deep in his pockets, his back bent nearly double, and his head hung low on his chest, lifted up the right corner of his mouth and smiled a greeting to all.

In history, as well as in Kafka's story, the public loses interest in fasting. There is not much to see, after all, and other entertainments take its place. Kafka's hunger artist becomes a minor attraction in a large circus. In the story's conclusion, the faster in his self-imposed cage is finally allowed to go without food for as long as he wants. In truth, he has been forgotten, hidden in a nest of straw, until a few moments before his death. At this time, he asks for forgiveness and confesses, "I always wanted you to admire my fasting." The amiable circus manager assures him they *do* admire him. The hunger artist protests they should not, since fasting came so easily and his reasons for fasting were not profound. "I couldn't find the food I liked," the dying man whispers. "If I had found it, believe me, I should have made no fuss and stuffed myself like you or anyone else."

The circus manager replaces the hunger artist with a young panther. Everyone loves the healthy, vibrant animal, who eats whatever is given to him, and who "seemed not even to miss his freedom; his noble body, furnished almost to the bursting point with all it needed, carried freedom around with it too." Now the audience crowds around the panther's cage and "the joy of life streamed with such ardent passion from his throat that for the onlookers it was not easy to stand the shock of it."

Most of us identify with the panther, not the hunger artist. Eating is something we think about when we wake up, before we go to bed, and many times in-between. Food is life. Life is freedom. Even the constraints of life are freedom.

Yet the opposite is also true. Perhaps a billion people in the world are overweight (as many can be described as hungry) and obesity often leads to a constrained life: diabetes, high blood pressure, heart attacks. Food is our enemy, and so we walk the aisles of supermarkets searching for ice cream that is not really ice cream, for pockets of flavored air, taste without calories.

Food fascinates us. Yet the opposite is also true. Hunger fascinates us.

A few years after Franz Kafka wrote "A Hunger Artist," there was a brief resurgence of the form. In 1926, in Berlin, six hunger artists exhibited at the same time. One performance took place in a popular restaurant where in the middle of the

hall, under a glass bell, a man in a dinner jacket smoked cigarettes and sipped water. A nearby blackboard announced that he
had not eaten for twenty-eight days. As one newspaper reported, "Around him corpulent gentlemen and fashionably
dressed ladies are consuming Wiener Schnitzel with fried potatoes. They are discussing whether the hunger record will be
broken this time."

In 2003, an American magician lived without food for forty-
four days in a six foot by six foot by three foot box strung up in
the air near Tower Bridge in London. The entertainer, David
Blaine, had done endurance tricks before—encasing himself in
a block of ice and being buried alive in a glass coffin. Now he
was the century's first hunger artist. The response was mixed.
An estimated quarter million people visited the site to see a
man sit and do nothing. Some women held banners declaring
their love and support. Others ran naked under the box. Some
men said David Blaine was a hero. Some called him an idiot.
On the street below, members of the crowd pelted the box with
rotten eggs, taunted Blaine with the smell of sizzling hamburg-
ers, and organized a movement to keep him awake at night with
drums and foghorns. They showed a surprising degree of anger
and distaste. A hundred years had passed since the heyday of
hunger artists like Giovanni Succi. In that time, television had
brought famine into our living rooms, and the bodies of starving
women and children—especially children—had become familiar to us. In that time, too, we came to revere the hunger striker,
cultural icons like Mahatma Gandhi, who used his hunger to
further peace and religious tolerance. Even as David Blaine
fasted for entertainment, other people were fasting for social
justice in Turkey, in Chile, in China, in the United States.

Some ten thousand people gathered to witness the end of Blaine's forty-four-day fast and many more watched on television. The newspapers described a carnival atmosphere with food and souvenir vendors, cries and gasps from the girls, songs, and flags. The door to the box opened, and soon Blaine was explaining to the crowd how he had learned to appreciate the simple things in life: a sunset, a smile. He had learned how strong we are as human beings. He had learned how necessary it is to have a sense of humor, to laugh at everything because nothing makes sense.

"This has been the most important experience of my life," he said, weeping. "I love you all."

. . .

In the annals of fasting, forty-four days is unimpressive. In June of 1965, a twenty-seven-year-old man, known as Mr. A. B., presented himself to physicians at the University Department of Medicine in Dundee, Scotland. He weighed 456 pounds. "Initially," reads the resulting paper in the *Postgraduate Medical Journal*, "there was no intention of making his fast a protracted one." But the young man adapted so well and was so "eager to reach his ideal weight," and the days passed, and his medical signs were normal, and more days passed, and still he persisted—drinking only as much water as he wanted, along with a daily vitamin pill—and more days passed, and then somehow a year had gone by, and then more than a year.

At first Mr. A. B. stayed in the university hospital. Rather soon, he was allowed to go home and return every day to have his urine collected and vital signs checked. The researchers took blood samples every two weeks. From Day 93 to Day 162, Mr. A. B. got potassium supplements. From Day 345 to Day 355, he was given sodium. His blood sugar, or glucose level, dropped quite low, yet Mr. A. B. "felt well and walked about normally" without any symptoms of hypoglycemia. His weight loss averaged .72 pounds a day. That sustained loss, the low level of blood sugar, and the results of other tests convinced the scientists that their patient was not secretly eating. Eventually, during the course of 382 days without food, he lost 276 pounds. Five years after the fast, he had only gained back sixteen.

He must, at times, have felt like a god. He lived like a tree, a rowan or oak, on air and sunshine. He lived more like spirit than matter. Did he try and walk through walls? Did he think of himself as a ghost?

We do not, of course, know what this young man felt or thought during those thirteen months. The *Postgraduate Medical Journal* says only, at the end, "We wish to express our gratitude to Mr. A. B. for his cheerful cooperation and steadfast application to the task of achieving a normal physique." The citation in the 1971 *Guinness Book of Records* briefly gives his name and poundage. Soon afterward, Guinness stopped recording long fasts because of the dangers involved.

. . .

When I was nineteen, I wanted to be a writer. My friend Stephanie also wanted to be a writer. We wanted to know the truth. That's what we thought writing was about. Stephanie and I sat at my kitchen table, perhaps drinking tea, perhaps making sandwiches, and I remember her declaring with emphasis, "I always write better when I'm hungry." I disagreed, although I didn't say so. Hunger only made me want to eat. Still, I knew what she meant in the larger sense: artists shouldn't be too comfortable. Artists need hunger as a verb. They need to desire. Moreover, in my time and place, in 1973 in Berkeley, California, the role of art was to stand outside established powers and successes, outside the state, outside capitalism—outside satiety.

It is not new, this portrait of the artist as a hungry young man. In 1890, Knut Hamsun published his autobiographical novel *Hunger.* What we know about the physiology of hunger matches up surprisingly well with his description. The unnamed narrator survives for weeks and months on insufficient food, moving from lodging to lodging, sometimes sleeping in the street, often walking the street in a kaleidoscope of moods, talking to himself, and scribbling out the articles that bring him a few kroners so he can repeat the cycle of a hurried meal and semi-starvation. In this story, hunger is all about emotion. The narrator is under siege to his own attacks of rage or fancy. We are introduced to him in the middle of his hunger and so we can never say we know the whole man, for we only catch glimpses of someone in a storm, his attributes exaggerated, overly conscientious, overly sensitive, now frantic, now furious, always self-absorbed.

Often enough, he is euphoric, a condition many fasters describe, "I had arrived at the joyful insanity hunger was; I was empty and free of pain." Or "I was drunk with starvation, my hunger had made me intoxicated. . . . I lay in a state of utter absence from myself and felt deliciously out of it."

Sometimes, his senses are unnaturally acute. He is aware of every sight, every sound, every smell, and they all seem meaningful: the brown dog and its silver collar, the maid with her sleeves rolled up. Details overwhelm him, and the world "poured into me with a staggering distinctness as if a strong light had fallen on everything." Without warning, this clarity tips into mysticism, the state of no-mind, "as though my brains simply ran quietly out of my head and left me empty."

But hunger is hardly a friend. In scene after scene, the narrator weeps or vomits or curses God. He falls into depression. He betrays his ideals. He bullies an old cake seller. The hunger in his stomach gnaws "without mercy . . . like a couple of dozen tiny creatures who put their heads over to one side . . . then put their heads over to the other side."

At the end of the novel, feverish and ill, the narrator is taken on as a worker aboard a ship. Just like that, he sails away from the city, away from hunger. This was a ten-year pattern in Knut Hamsun's own life, periods of physical labor mixed with the poverty of the struggling writer. The book *Hunger* was his entrance into success and the end of that struggle. Critics would later describe Hamsun's willingness to be hungry as a drive toward creativity. In his discussion of the novel, poet Robert Bly believes that hunger leads the narrator to psychic health: "Somehow his unconscious has chosen this suffering as a way for some part of him to get well. The hero of *Hunger* obeys the unconscious and remains in hunger, despite suffering, until he has lived through what he must or learned what he had to."

In the 1933 novel *Down and Out in Paris and London*, George Orwell tried and failed to shake up the mythology of the starving artist. The story is clearly autobiographical, the adventures of a poor student in Paris who discovers "the boredom which is inseparable from poverty; the times when you have nothing to do and, being underfed, can interest yourself in nothing." Later, Orwell's character spends a day in bed reading *The Memoirs of Sherlock Holmes*. "It was all that I felt equal to, without food. Hunger reduces one to an utterly spineless, brainless condition. . . . It is as though one has been turned into a jellyfish, or as though one's blood has been pumped out and luke-warm water substituted."

The effect of all this complaining, however, with its literary allusions, is only to strengthen the central glamour: hunger as a rite of passage. Hunger has always been seen as a unique form of suffering that can lead to insight, both in art and religion. Asceticism brings us closer to our version of God. The monks in their monasteries, the artists in their garrets—they grow lean and leaner and more spiritual and more artistic. That may have been Kafka's joke at the end: all his faster wanted was better food, not the truth, not a deeper understanding of life, but a desire for more than what life can offer.

. . .

Hunger is finally about death. We are fascinated by hunger because after 50 days or 90 days or 382 days, hunger ends in a body forced to cannibalize itself. Death is a major theme in our own life, too, the conclusion we are sliding toward. Death is the real story.

For a time in my life, I became something of a hunger artist, collecting news clippings about starvation and famine, labeling folders Somalia and Ethiopia. A billion people in the world were hungry. Even children in America were hungry. My impetus did not seem to be about death, but birth. I was thirty years old and pregnant. A gate opened inside me with a neat and nearly audible hormonal click. It was the gate to grief, not sentimentalism exactly, but something that might have veered close. Certainly that gate swung open at any sentimental cue—a country-western song, a photograph, a sad movie. I couldn't understand why children were dying because they had no food. I gave birth to my daughter and fed her my body. Later, I had a son and he, too, drank from me. I was feeding the world. This was not aggrandizement so much as myth. At the center of our life, we are Eve or Prometheus or Odysseus. At the center of my life, I fed the world, and yet children were dying.

This lasted for a few years. I would sit in a fast-food restaurant with my five-year-old son. He was here for the toy they had set like bait in a circle of french fries, orange soda, and meat. As I read the newspaper, I saw the picture of a hungry child in our most recent famine. The gate swung open. I knew because I had made it my business to know what was happening to this child. The fat in her tissues had been used up long ago, so that her skin looked loose and her eyes sunk into bone. Her brain needed glucose of which the only source now was her own protein. Already the digestive enzymes in her stomach and pancreas had been sacrificed. Soon she would eat the muscles in her arms, in her legs, in her heart.

Where I sat at the table, I could see the restaurant's playground. Small children bounced up and down on brightly colored plastic. I wanted to snatch this little girl from the page, hold her, raise her, send her to college. My sight blurred and instinctively, immediately, I pushed hard against the gate. This grief, whose was it? *This was not my baby*. I did not burst out crying. I did not frighten my son in the middle of the fast-food restaurant. Instead, I assembled his cardboard prize and turned to another page of the newspaper. I felt tired, but only deep down, so far down it was hardly noticeable.

Most of us know this exhaustion. We are afraid that the pain of other people will subtract the joy from our life, that our joy will be impossible next to their pain. A child dying of hunger cannot be juxtaposed. A child dying because she has no food does not make sense. She shatters the view from the kitchen window. She shatters your son's first day at school. Eventually I stopped collecting famine stories. I shut the gate. But I never turned the lock.

. . .

A little hunger, scientists are beginning to say, is good for us. We would live longer and be healthier if we were hungrier. In animals, and probably in humans, reducing the daily intake of calories by 30 percent can mean lower blood pressure, lower cholesterol levels, resistance to cancer and Alzheimer's disease, and a longer life span. The National Institute on Aging has recently given out a series of multi-million-dollar grants to study calorie restriction in adult men and women.

Informal work has already begun. The Calorie Restriction Society is a group of enthusiasts who list over 150 members on their website. Many members have cut their daily consumption by 25 percent, keeping all the protein, carbohydrates, fats, vitamins, and minerals they need for a nutritious diet. Men over six feet tall, weighing approximately 175 pounds, will eat 1,500–1,900 calories a day. Other calorie-restrictors eat less. Typical calorie-restrictors tend to be introverted, self-disciplined, and male. They admit that their lifestyles can lead to obsessive behaviors, which they try to avoid. Their goal is to live longer, not less well. They admit that calorie restriction can mean a reduced sex drive and greater sensitivity to cold, although they also point to feelings of vitality and increased mental awareness. Most say that hunger is a constant companion. They share strategies to reduce their cravings for food as they map out their days and meals in a war against hunger. They are the newest version of the hunger artist, happy to be in a good fight.

Periodic fasting may be as good or better than reducing calories. In a 2003 study, mice were fasted every other day and then allowed to eat freely. They maintained a stable weight and had lower blood glucose and insulin levels than the control group, which meant a reduced risk of diabetes and heart disease. Outside the laboratory, people have long promoted fasting for health. Hippocrates recommended fasting, as did Plato. Mark Twain wrote, "A little starvation can really do more for the average sick man than can the best of medicines and the best doctors." Around the world, clinics supervise therapeutic fasts—that period of time in which an individual can safely abstain from food, living like an oak or rowan, calmly drinking water, resting and reading, sunbathing just a little. Some patients fast for as long as thirty days. They fast because they have rheumatoid arthritis or stomach problems or high blood pressure. They fast because they are diabetic or overweight. They believe they are accelerating the natural healing powers of the body. A number of these people seem to get better. (A small percentage of people with metabolic diseases should not fast at all, for any length of time or any reason. Unfortunately, you do not always know if this applies to you.)

What happens in your body after twelve hours without food, after eighteen hours, after seventy-two hours, after seven days, after thirty days? What happens when you just eat less? What happens during months and years of malnutrition and semi-starvation? We understand less than it seems we should. On the subject of hunger, so everyday, so deadly, we have surprising gaps of knowledge. We begin the twenty-first century with renewed interest.

Hunger is as big as history. Some four thousand years ago, an inscription on the tomb of the Egyptian Ankhtifi read, "All of upper Egypt was dying of hunger to such a degree that everyone had come to eating his children." The Bible is full of stories about hunger. Two-thirds of the population of Italy starved to death in 1347. A potato fungus triggered the Great Hunger of Ireland in 1845–50, which killed a million people and is still commemorated by monuments, websites, and re-created voyages of the "coffin ships" that brought Irish emigrants to North America. Seven million people died in 1919–21 from a famine in the Ukraine and southwestern Russia. Four million died in the Bengal famine of 1943–44. The largest known famine killed over thirty million Chinese from 1958–62.

Hunger is as intimate as self. It is what I feel before lunch. It is how I think about my body, my breasts, my thighs. My mother went hungry during the Great Depression, and I am partly who I am because of that. I am largely who I am because I do *not* experience involuntary hunger. I am who I am because of the specific way hunger affects my cells—an efficient response to insulin, decisive actions by the liver. I have been shaped by hunger, and I have adapted to hunger. Like a hibernating bear, I can live off my fat. I could live for forty days in a box. In the complexity of being human, I might use this ability to make money, get closer to Jesus, or convince the British to leave India. I shape hunger too.

Every morning we wake up hungry. Hunger and satiety are two poles we swing between all our life. Hunger is traveling in our bloodstream now. Hunger is clanging the bell of the hypothalamus. Hunger is driving us into the kitchen. We are in the passenger's seat. We are all hunger artists.

EIGHTEEN HOURS

THINK HARD ABOUT SPAGHETTI. THE IMAGE IN your mind begins the process of digestion. A commercial for the Olive Garden sends a chemical message from your cerebral cortex to your nerve cells in the lower brain, which in turn sends a message to the stomach and pancreas, stimulating their production of enzymes, acids, and mucus. The lower brain also pulls the alarm at the salivary glands. Your mouth starts to water. As you debate—the red or white sauce, potato salad, a glass of Chardonnay—hormones move through your bloodstream and prompt cells to release fatty acids, which will be converted into the energy needed to digest your food. Your pancreas secretes insulin, another hormone that will help turn the digested food into more energy. Long before the waitress comes to the table, your body has been primed.

Even earlier, a hormone produced in your empty stomach may have been sent to the appetite centers in the lower brain, prompting your interest in commercials about spaghetti, prompting the digestive wheels to start rolling. Eating is the house that Jack built, a series of inter-reactions.

You take a bite and start to chew. In the back of your throat, vaporized molecules of pasta reach the olfactory cells in your nose through the same passage that allows for nasal drip. The sensation of tomatoes and basil is really a mix of taste and smell. This mix stimulates the release of more free fatty acids into the bloodstream and more secretions of digestive juices and insulin. Meanwhile, your saliva contains an enzyme that is splitting starches into sugars, enhancing the sensation of sweetness. Saliva also stimulates taste receptors, lubricates food, cleanses your mouth, and is weakly antibacterial. Once you decide to stop chewing, you tongue your food back. In terms of digestion, this movement is your last conscious act.

A swallowing reflex sends food down into the throat, where muscles contract and relax to push it farther down into the esophagus, where muscles contract and relax to push it into the stomach. A gateway keeps the contents from being regurgitated. Now the stomach is turning like a slow blender as muscular waves mix the food in an acidic environment strong enough to dissolve metal. The wine you drank is absorbed immediately by blood vessels in the stomach wall and sent to circulate throughout your system, as are a few salts, water, and molecules of glucose already broken down from the carbohydrates in your meal. Everything else is further mixed and mashed into a semi-liquid, pushed down toward the small intestine, and stored until the intestine is ready to receive it, squirt by squirt, through another tightly controlled gateway.

Soon—even though it will be hours before all your food is turned into the molecules your cells can use—you need to stop eating. You need to feel satisfied. The stretching of the stomach sends a signal through the nervous system to suppress the appetite center in the lower brain. The stomach and pancreas send additional hormones to the brain with the same message. Scientists speculate that your mouth with its chewing, salivating, tasting, and swallowing may also be metering the food. After enough chews, your mouth signals stop.

You also stop out of habit. This is the amount you ate at your last meal, and your sense of convention will prevent you from eating more and from eating again for the next few hours. In a study done with two severely amnesic patients—men who could not remember events that had happened only a few moments ago, who could not remember that they were involved in an experiment, who could not remember the faces of the people who brought them food every day—memory played a surprising role. On three separate occasions, both patients readily ate a second meal ten to thirty minutes after their first one and then attempted a third dinner. The food, after all, looked good, and they had no memory, no habit, to constrain them.

The small intestine does most of the work of absorbing nutrients, its inner walls lined with thousands of circular folds with millions of fingerlike projections that secrete mucus and split complex molecules into simpler ones. As the stomach empties its contents of food, its motions slow. The small intestine speeds up. More enzymes are sent in from the pancreas and liver. Now the organs are talking to each other in a cascade of hormones and reflexes: less of this, more of that, *go, go, go.*

The digestive system does so much signaling, with such verve and independence, that it has been called "the second brain" by Dr. Michael Gershon, who helped discover the field of neurogastroenterology and who is prone to such remarks as "a renaissance of the gut is underway" and "it is morning in the abdomen." The nervous system in the stomach and intestines contains more nerve cells than the spinal cord and is able to work entirely on its own, without help from the brain: sending, receiving, coordinating messages, initiating reflexes, processing sensory data, and acting on that information.

The walls of the gut must allow certain molecules—the broken-down products of carbohydrates, protein, and fat (but not bacteria)—to pass out, into the body, while they prevent the body itself from passing into the hollow spaces of the stomach and intestines. "Paradoxical as it may seem," Gershon writes, "the gut is a tunnel that permits the exterior to run right through us. Whatever is in the lumen of the gut is actually outside of our bodies." If you bleed into the pouch of your stomach, you can bleed to death. Similarly, water and food that move through the bowel without being absorbed is the same as not drinking or eating at all.

Your meal at the Olive Garden is largely made of carbohydrates, which range from single sugar units to chains of starches. Within thirty minutes of mixing with the juices in the small intestine, almost all the starches in your pasta have been converted into forms of glucose, a simple sugar. That's the point. For much of the body, glucose is the preferred fuel. Within a cell, glucose molecules are split into carbon dioxide and water, a process that releases energy that the cell needs to function: to transport material across a membrane or to move in a way that moves something larger, like the muscles in your heart. Except under extraordinary conditions, the brain, retina, and gonads run solely on glucose.

In the intestinal walls, glucose molecules pass into tiny blood vessels that empty into a large vein that connects to the liver where the blood is cleansed. From the liver, glucose is sent out into the bloodstream, celebratory. The hormone insulin now helps move glucose into the cells that need it. Excess glucose is stored in the liver in a form called glycogen. Muscle tissue can also store small amounts of glycogen to be used for bursts of exercise. When the liver and muscle cells are full, the remaining glucose is converted and stored as fat. One hour after eating a meal, the level of glucose in your blood is relatively high. Two or three hours after that, the level is usually back to normal.

You also had protein in your meal—anchovies in the antipasto, prosciutto on the caramelized pears. Proteins are amino acids arranged in different patterns. They make up three-quarters of the solid parts of the body, our rafters and floors, trusses and ceilings, the stuff of muscles as well as enzymes, hormones, and antibodies. We manufacture nine of the twenty amino acids needed for growth and metabolism. We must eat the rest. In the small intestine, long chains of amino acids are split into smaller chains, which can pass into blood vessels and on to the liver. The liver will convert excess amino acids into glucose or glycogen.

Fats are made of fatty acids and glycerol (similar to a simple sugar). In the small intestine, bile from the liver breaks down fat globules so pancreatic enzymes can act on them. Fatty acids enter the cells of the intestinal lining and are transported into the lymph system. From there they go into the blood, the liver, and back into the bloodstream. Like glucose, fatty acids are broken down by cells to produce energy, more than double the energy we get from glucose and the main energy used by muscles during the day. Fat is easily stored in tissues, which also serve as heat insulation. As the body requires more fatty acids, they are released from stored fat. This happens at an extraordinary rate: half the fatty acids in the blood are being used and replaced by new fatty acids every two to three minutes. Unlike carbohydrates and protein, fatty acids cannot be converted into glucose.

As your meal is disassembled and absorbed, it is being moved toward and into the large intestine. At that point, all the nutrients have been diverted into the blood or lymph system. What remain are water, indigestible roughage, waste, and bacteria. The colon's job is to reabsorb the water. Otherwise, we would dehydrate.

By now, dinner was many hours ago. Your intestines keep working. Your stomach notices it is empty. The stomach produces hunger hormones such as ghrelin, which is sent up to the lower brain. Ghrelin has a Dickensian personality, a thin and pathetic Oliver Twist: "Please, sir, can I have more gruel?" When mice are injected with ghrelin, they eat enormous amounts of food and gain weight. When human volunteers are injected with ghrelin, they go to the buffet table and eat 30 percent more than anyone else at the buffet. In lean or normal-weight humans, ghrelin levels rise just before a meal and then go down, up and down through the course of the day. In one animal study, a high-fat diet decreased ghrelin production, a prompt for the body to eat less, and a low-protein diet increased ghrelin, a prompt for the body to eat more. Ghrelin levels are consistently higher in dieters after they have lost weight, and they are near their highest in patients with anorexia nervosa (who live with and ignore that signal).

Another hormone in the system tells the brain how much fat you already have. Leptin is made by fat cells. If you have put on weight, the higher level of leptin nudges the brain to listen more closely to signals of satiety. If you have lost weight, lower levels of leptin encourage the brain to eat more. The overweight body soon adapts to a high level of leptin, however, perhaps by becoming resistant to its signal. Overweight humans often have low levels of ghrelin, too, another "I'm not hungry" signal that is not being heard. These dysfunctions may be adaptations, part of a genetic heritage or "thrifty gene syndrome" that allow people to hoard fat and stay alive during periods of food shortage.

Philosophers call the domain your food enters the "recessive body," an interior world we cannot see and do not fully understand. Our feelings about this world are understandably mixed. We are glad not to be in charge. We welcome the body's competence even as we are intimidated by it. As Lewis Thomas wrote, "If I were informed tomorrow that I was in direct communication with my liver, and could now take over, I would become deeply depressed. I'd sooner be told, forty thousand feet over Denver, that the 747 jet in which I had a coach seat was now mine to operate. . . . I am unconstitutionally unable to make hepatic decisions and I prefer not to be obliged to, ever."

If we are not in charge, who is? The answer may be everything: the cerebral cortex, the circulatory system, the respiratory system, the pancreas, the intestinal walls, the nerves, the muscles, the hormones, the taste of an apple, the word for apple, the memory of an apple. We are a gestalt. Aristotle called us the "ensouled body," the body living and lived. Neurobiologist Antonio Damasio reminded us sharply, "The self is a repeatedly reconstructed biological state; it is *not* a little person, the infamous homunculus, inside your brain contemplating what is going on."

The construction and reconstruction of self requires a constant transformation of the world. We take in chunks of matter and break them down into smaller parts and then into smaller parts still, molecules of glucose or fatty acids, and then we break those down further into the energy our cells need. We deconstruct the world, and we build it up, creating tissue and bone, movement and thought. Then we use thought to do this again, over and over, many times a day, every day.

. . .

You eat your spaghetti around seven p.m., go to bed early, and fall asleep. You wake, urinate, brush your teeth. You haven't eaten for twelve hours. Hormones are circulating through your bloodstream, from the stomach to the brain, from the brain to the stomach. Your body tugs at your sleeve. It is time for breakfast. What looks good?

Appetite can intertwine with hunger and then separate. You have an appetite for ice cream although you are not really hungry. You may be hungry for food without the appetite for anything specific. Appetite is desire, born of biology, molded by experience and culture. In the morning, you want bacon and eggs, toast with butter, a glass of orange juice—the breakfast you associate with abundance. You want mango yogurt, something light and exotic. You want fiber. You want your grandmother's golden, dollar-sized pancakes—the breakfast you associate with love. Actually you don't want anything yet, just a cup of coffee with cream and sugar. You want a croissant. You want small objects dyed in lime-green and purple, a bowl of Trix. You want cooked tomatoes and bits of kidney. You want your traditional meal of miso soup, broiled fish, steamed rice, pickled vegetable, and green tea. You want a yam. You want salt. You want whale blubber. Commonly, I have a slice of apple pie.

When appetite and satiety conflict, appetite often wins. We know this whenever we leave the table after that stomach-distending holiday meal. We recognize it in most banana splits. We see it in patients being fed nutrients through a tube; their hunger is abated but their appetite remains, and they will secretly eat solid food even at the risk of pain or vomiting.

Appetite's alter ego is aversion. When aversion and hunger conflict, aversion often wins. We won't eat a breakfast that doesn't appeal to us. We lose weight traveling in a country with unfamiliar food. We pass up the appetizer that has a strange texture or smell. Our suspicion of food is an omnivore's defense, a conservative force, and we share it with all kinds of small mammals. A calm state of mind can help us overcome this neophobia. When psychologists had subjects play a boring video game, a neutral video game, and an exciting video game before selecting a snack, the boring video game was followed by more food adventurousness and the exciting game by less.

Like many emotions, aversion can go straight to the stomach. If you once suffered food poisoning after a tuna sandwich, you may reject tuna for a long time. You may feel sick eating something you define as disgusting or morally wrong. In a study of Jews who followed kosher dietary laws, half felt nauseated at the idea of eating pork or a meat-dairy combination. Even vomiting, a dramatic and reverse movement of the stomach, can begin with a disturbing thought. In extreme situations, when men and women are starving to death, they may still conform to social taboos. Cannibalism is not a common response to hunger or famine. The majority of us will die before we eat human flesh. People with anorexia nervosa are also paying more attention to their emotional needs (which may have a biological basis) than their body's hunger. Although they may feel hunger acutely, their appetite, their aversion is more important.

It is time for breakfast and what looks good to you, the synergy of your appetite and aversion, is unique. But let's say instead that the phone rings. There is a message from work. You have to leave, right now. You can eat later.

We will have varying responses to skipping a meal, based on our metabolism and psychology. In a few hours, as the level of our blood sugar continues to drop, we might also experience a drop in energy. That might make us anxious or irritable. We might develop a headache. We might have a gnawing sensation below our rib cage. We might rumble embarrassingly. Who knew the body could make such sounds? Borborygmus is the onomatopoeia for the increased activity of the intestines as they squeeze every bit of old material through, all the way to the rectum, causing the collision of water and air pockets, bubbles, and gurgles. We might feel some mild cramping. To be hungry is to be uncomfortable, and most of us experience hunger in the same way we experience pain, as a signal to do something.

Then again, we may hardly notice the fact that we haven't eaten since last night. Hunger has been pushed aside by busyness, the demands of a phone call. Or we may notice our hunger and feel unconcerned, even proud. To hunger a little is not a bad thing. Literally, hunger is the best sauce. We will enjoy our lunch more for being deprived of breakfast.

The philosopher Drew Leder called digestion "intermittent impressions in a shroud of absence." That's a fair description. Leder also wrote, "Hunger is experienced not just in abdominal ache but as a heaviness in the limbs, a yearning in the mouth."

You haven't eaten for over eighteen hours. It is almost noon. Your biological clock knows the time. Your body understands, even if you don't, that it needs two hundred grams of glucose a day. Your brain wants at least half of that. The level of glucose in your bloodstream is low. The level of ghrelin in your bloodstream is high, an insistent knocking at the brain stem's door. You feel that insistence as emotion. Suddenly all other concerns fall away. You focus on lunch. You feel a yearning in your mouth.

THIRTY-SIX HOURS

W HEN ANGELO DEL PARIGI, A RESEARCH FELLOW at the National Institute of Diabetes and Digestive and Kidney Diseases, wants to do a study, he puts an ad in the newspapers and waits and hopes. In 2001, Angelo needed a group of men and a matched group of women who did not have a family history of obesity or diabetes; who did not have a personal history of substance abuse or addiction; who did not suffer from claustrophobia, depression, psychosis, anorexia nervosa, or bulimia nervosa; who had no dietary restrictions; who had had a minimum of radiation exposure; who had not taken medication for the last month; who did not have any metal in their bodies; and who could be taken from their lives and sent to live for over a week at the Clinical Diabetes and Nutrition Section of the National Institutes of Health in Phoenix, Arizona. It's not as easy as announcing a garage sale or finding that special used car. The ad promised the subjects a free medical checkup and reimbursement for their time. Angelo is not allowed to say how much reimbursement. The ad also mentioned a thirty-six-hour fast.

Lots of people called. Few qualified. In the end, twenty-two men and twenty-two women were shown their living quarters—a ward with five bedrooms, a TV room, a large kitchen run by hospital staff, and a series of doors leading to laboratories and machines. The décor was strictly medical. The subjects watched a video and signed a consent form.

The object of the study was to see if the brains of men and women responded differently to short-term hunger and satiation. For seven days, the subjects ate a weight-maintaining diet of 50 percent carbohydrates, 30 percent fat, and 20 percent protein. Then one morning, no breakfast was served and nothing again all day. The next morning, after thirty-six hours without food, the subjects were taken to a room and asked to lie still while Angelo scanned their brain using positron emission tomography, a mapping of the cerebral blood flow that reveals which areas are being activated. A plastic feeding tube was inserted into the subject's mouth to the middle of the tongue, and water was sent through the tube to induce swallowing before each scan. This had been practiced before so patients could become familiar with the procedure. They had also chosen the flavor of their future liquid meal—strawberry, chocolate, or vanilla. The first two scans were the baseline: a hungry subject, with tube on tongue. The tests took a minute each. After each scan, the subjects rated their feelings of hunger and satiety, and blood samples were collected to measure glucose, free fatty acids, insulin, leptin, and other hormones. The next two scans measured responses after the subject had been given a taste of the liquid meal. The last two scans were given after the subject had been fed a liquid meal for twenty-five minutes: a satiated man or woman now, with tube on tongue.

When you stop eating, you start using your stored calories, your savings bank. Typically, 85 percent of those calories are in fat. Another 14 percent are in protein. The remaining 1 percent is in the form of carbohydrates, circulating as glucose through the blood system or stashed in the liver and muscles as glycogen. An average-sized man might have 141,000 calories stored in fat tissue, 24,000 calories stored in muscle mass, and 300 calories stored in glycogen. Theoretically, that will last 80 days at 2,000 calories a day. The weak link is obvious. Most of the energy your body needs can now come from fatty acids. But your brain, your eyes, and your gonads still require glucose. And you don't have much.

In the first twenty-four hours of fasting, the level of glucose in your bloodstream drops slightly, which causes a decline in circulating insulin. The low level of insulin stimulates fat tissues to release free fatty acids that travel in the bloodstream to the liver, where the process of fat metabolism starts. The decrease in insulin also stimulates the secretion of a hormone that raises blood sugar levels by promoting glucose production. Obligingly, your liver starts converting its supply of glycogen until it is gone, usually in a day. Triglycerides are chains of fatty acids bound with a molecule of glycerol. The liver can convert this glycerol into small amounts of glucose, too. The lactate or lactic acid in your muscles can also be re-synthesized back into glucose.

The new hormonal environment causes more amino acids to be released by muscle tissue and sent to the liver and kidneys to be converted to glucose as well. By thirty-six hours, the second day of your fast, your production of glucose will rely heavily on this use of protein. At this point, the body's goal is to avoid using glucose as much as possible and to produce the glucose the brain needs from bits of this or that—mostly from muscle tissue.

In Angelo Del Parigi's experiment, men and women did not show any significant differences in how they rated feelings of hunger and satiety. There were no differences in the appetite center in the lower brain, which regulates the balance between hunger and satiety and its effect on body weight. There were no differences in the chemical and hormonal signals sent through the blood, except for lower levels in women of a hormone that inhibits hunger. But hungry men had more activity than women in the area of the brain that processes emotion, as if they *felt* their hunger more acutely. And satiated men had more activity than women in the part of the brain that processes the association between stimulus and response, in short, the feeling of satisfaction: *hey, that was good!* Satiated women had more activity than men in the occipital temporal cortex, the seat of object recognition. No one knows yet what this means.

Not just once, but many times, Angelo has asked people not to eat so he can watch their brains light up. Other experiments with thirty-six hours of fasting were between lean and obese men and lean and obese women. Obese individuals responded to satiation with greater activity in their prefrontal cortex, an area associated with complex thought and the inhibition of "inappropriate response tendencies" and decreased activity in the lower brain area associated with emotion. Does this suggest that obese people respond to eating and satiation with more social and cognitive inhibitions, perhaps learned and acquired? Do they get less emotional reward from eating? Again, we don't know, and Angelo won't speculate.

On one level, Angelo Del Parigi is like any medieval cartographer, purely obsessed with filling in the blank spaces. Here is a mountain we hadn't seen before. Here are the headwaters of the great rushing river. Here is a map of the world, in this case, the human brain.

But these studies are also practical. Women suffer more from obesity and eating disorders than men, so it is useful to know if there are gender differences in how women and men respond to hunger. For people trying to diet, it is useful to know how they will react to calorie deprivation and weight loss. The problems associated with obesity make it one of the biggest health threats of the twenty-first century, on the World Health Organization's top ten list, on the top five list for developed countries. The morbidly obese can suffer horribly. Even the mildly obese risk shorter lives.

"In terms of treatment, obesity is so much harder to deal with than malnutrition," Angelo says. "In malnutrition, there is a deficiency, and we deal with that deficiency. Obesity is more complex."

It is not just about health. It is also about money. Over half the adults in the United States are considered overweight or obese; the same is true for Mexico, Brazil, Chile, Colombia, Peru, Uruguay, Paraguay, Russia, Finland, England, Bulgaria, Morocco, and Saudi Arabia. One researcher described this as an "epidemic of energy storage." An epidemic requires a cure—a vaccine or drug. All those cures translate into a lot of customers.

In 1994, when researchers at Rockefeller University injected synthesized leptin into fat mice, the mice slimmed down immediately, losing almost all their fat and none of their muscle mass. Human volunteers for the next phase of the study were easy to find. Before the trials began, Rockefeller University held a silent auction for drug companies interested in the "rights" to leptin and got a twenty-million-dollar down payment, with a possible hundred million in total installments.

Leptin did not prove to be the magic pill. In the first experiment with seventy-three overweight subjects, only forty-three completed the study. The rest complained of side effects like extreme skin irritation. Natural levels of leptin also vary among individuals, and the response to more leptin was erratic. Of those receiving the highest dosage, some people gained twelve pounds while others lost thirty.

We keep hitting the same brick wall: the human body defends itself vigorously against weight loss. Moreover, energy maintenance is intertwined with other functions. Ghrelin does not only make us hungry, but it is also essential for tissue repair, bone strength, and muscle growth. It may not be a good idea to suppress it. Knocking out a brain neurotransmitter that controls appetite might also skew the one that regulates blood pressure. Like a good watch, the biochemistry of metabolism is not something we want just anyone to take apart.

Many scientists are optimistic. In the last ten years, they have learned an enormous amount, and within ten years, some expect to be able to control how people gain and lose weight. Importantly, the work on of leptin in 1994 led to renewed research in the chemistry of hunger.

Studies in leptin or ghrelin might also help patients with the loss of appetite and wasting found after surgery, in old age, and in illnesses like AIDS. In some cases, a drug need only stimulate the desire to eat. Cancer patients with wasting or cachexia, however, suffer the loss not only of fatty tissues but also of muscle and bone, reflecting an imbalance in their protein metabolism. When a cancer cachexia mouse model (a mouse injected with human melanoma cells) was given ghrelin, the wasting was reversed.

Obesity research has already benefited children with genetic mutations that cause them to eat uncontrollably. One eight-year-old weighed nearly two hundred pounds and had to use a wheel-chair. Her cousin reached sixty-five pounds at the age of two.

When their alarmed parents locked the cupboards, the children scavenged for garbage scraps and gnawed frozen fish sticks. Knowing that low levels of leptin encourage eating, a consulting doctor tried a blood test for leptin. The children had none. None at all. Their genes lacked the nucleic acid that codes for the hormone. In this case, leptin injections were miraculous, and the children are now in the range of normal weight.

Prader-Willi syndrome is another genetic disorder in which children show a desperate hunger for food. One boy wrote of "piranhas in the stomach." The stimulated appetite combines with a low metabolism to produce morbid obesity. Victims of Prader-Willi syndrome are often mildly retarded and suffer from repetitive obsessive behavior such as the hoarding of possessions. They have difficulty controlling their emotions. They have very high levels of ghrelin. Today many control their weight by living in group homes that supervise their eating. In the past, they regularly died before the age of thirty from an obesity-related disease. Some died from eating so much that their stomach stretched to its capacity and burst.

Angelo Del Parigi tells me that the same areas of the brain that light up when you are hungry also light up when you are thirsty, or in pain, or fighting for oxygen.

. . .

It has been thirty-six hours since you last ate food. You have used up your supply of glycogen and are now burning protein, little parts of yourself. Some intelligence in your stomach, your second brain, is outraged. You have a headache, as though your first brain, too, is protesting this idea. Your eyes are dry. You have a sharp pain behind one of them. You feel edgy. More than edgy. You don't care any more about the reimbursement or free medical checkup. You don't care about being nice to the doctors. You look forward to being fed strawberry-flavored liquid through a plastic tube.

. . .

Angelo Del Parigi induces short-term hunger as a way of exploring obesity. In fact, as we all know, short-term hunger is common in the world, although it does not usually mean a complete lack of food. This kind of hunger, linked to poverty, is also linked to obesity. Deprivation can cause overeating. When we skip a meal or go hungry for a day, the body gets alarmed—and then overcompensates. At the same time, low-fat foods like fresh vegetables and fruit are expensive and not often available in poor urban or rural stores. Less nutritious but high-caloric meals are cheaper, more convenient, and easier to prepare.

In America, over 30 million people—one in ten Americans—live in what is called food-insecure households. Twelve million of these are children. One in four people in line at a soup kitchen is a child. Most families that worry about food are headed by a single mother. A disproportionate number of families are Black or Hispanic. For the last four years, the number of households experiencing hunger has steadily increased.

In America, short-term hunger is a choice between paying for food at the end of the month and paying for rent or heat or medicine. It is a Sunday waiting for Monday and the school breakfast and lunch program. It is eating dry cereal for three days. It is shoplifting. It is being homeless or mentally ill or old.

In my home state of New Mexico, the Roadrunner Food Bank in Albuquerque distributes more than 50,000 pounds of food every day to hungry people. Part of the national Second Harvest program, the food bank gets salvageable products from donors, like large grocery stores, and redistributes them to a network of soup kitchens, day cares, group homes, and smaller food banks. The bank also purchases food in bulk. Their motto is, "The sooner you believe it, the sooner we can end it." In 2005, New Mexico led the nation in the percentage of people who have to worry about their next meal (almost 16 percent, or one in seven) and in the number of children who live below the poverty line (25 percent, or one in four). Almost half the people who get help from Roadrunner have a job. Often they work in service industries, as maids or waitresses, and can't stretch their paychecks to last a month.

The food bank has a new program that feeds kids over the weekend. Individual public schools identify which children seem to need more than the daily free breakfast and lunch and then sends them home with a backpack of food. Inside is a collection of single-serving, non perishable items: milk or juice in a box, raisins, beef stew or soup, animal crackers. Extra food is packed for pre-school siblings. Sometimes, when there are a lot of brothers and sisters at home, the backpack is so heavy that kindergartners and first graders have trouble carrying it. Some kids, naturally, sit down and start eating as soon as they are off school grounds. For that reason, the backpacks include a plastic spoon.

The director of Roadrunner gives backpacks of food to about 1,500 kids, and she commits to those kids throughout the school year. Summer is another story. Everyone in the hunger business knows that children go hungry in the summer.

From surveys and national reports, the director thinks that when there isn't enough food in the house, first adults skip meals, then older children. People turn to relatives, if possible. They thin the soup and make a box of macaroni last a long time. They wait it out.

At a Roadrunner Food Bank meeting, volunteers admit that their frustrations include the fear that they are enabling people. They see some fraud. They see some sloth. They see lots of dysfunction. While many Americans deny the existence of hunger in this country, others question the solution: if we give food away, if food is a basic right, what will motivate people to go out and work?

Unless you are living in the nineteenth century, the argument falls apart when you are faced with a six-year-old child. The director of the school backpack program shows me a drawing. The lines and splotches of brown and black don't mean much to me. Apparently the teacher in the class had the same problem, so she asked the little boy to explain. "This is a man," the child said, and the teacher dutifully wrote the words down, "who is angry because he just wants food."

It is not hard to believe that involuntary hunger also creates a new chemistry in the human body, metaphoric perhaps, or perhaps not, for shame is physical, frustration is physical. Hormone levels rise. Neurotransmitters spark. We don't have proof, but we can speculate: different areas of the brain light up when people are hungry because they have no choice.

SEVEN DAYS

IN AN ONLINE CHRISTIAN CHAT ROOM, A MAN discusses his three-day fast. He has a different kind of yearning—an appetite for God. Now he has not eaten for seventy-two hours, three days, what some people say is the hardest time. Mostly he feels empty, a sensation of odd-being more than ill. He is not hungry, and he sees that as a blessing. He has a bad taste in his mouth. He feels very tired. He feels a little weepy. Other people in this chat room have fasted, too, and he asks them for advice.

· · ·

The body responds to a lack of food by releasing fatty acids from stored fat. These are transported to the liver, which begins their breakdown into energy. The body also increases glucose production for the brain and other tissues that cannot use fatty acids. The liver empties its supply of glycogen and starts converting amino acids into glucose and urea. The kidneys also convert amino acids into glucose, with the byproduct of ammonia. Most of these amino acids are coming from muscle mass. Using up your protein, your muscles, your enzymes, and the structures of your cells cannot continue for long. Specifically, supplying the body's need for glucose in this way will end in death in two to three weeks.

The liver is our largest organ, about one fiftieth of the body's weight, glossy and dark red, capable of regenerating itself and sometimes called "the great chemical factory" for its ability to make so many things out of other things. The liver is a multi-tasker: filtering, cleansing, and storing blood; producing bile for digestion; producing blood-clotting agents; storing vitamins and iron; detoxing the system; storing and regulating glucose; synthesizing glucose from protein; and helping metabolize protein and fat.

By the third day of a fast, in the absence of incoming glucose, the liver begins to convert some fatty acids into compounds called ketone bodies. These can be used by cells that normally only use glucose. The brain has a barrier that blocks toxins in the bloodstream, as well as fats and fatty acids, but ketone bodies are allowed to slip through. The body is conserving protein by supplying the brain with a new fuel, a strategy unique to human beings and a few ruminants.

Ketone bodies sound like something in an auto shop: acetoacetic acid, beta-hydroxybutyric acid, and acetone. Scientists used to think the brain could not adapt from glucose to ketone bodies until after weeks of starvation. In fact, by the fourth day of a fast, as much as one-third of the brain's energy comes from ketones, the product of fatty acids. The brain and heart may actually run more efficiently on ketones than on glucose, in part because ketones provide more energy.

At the National Institutes of Health, Dr. Richard Veech calls ketone bodies "magic." They effectively mimic the work of insulin in the heart and brain, increase metabolic efficiency, may help cells deal better with trauma, and decrease the production of free radicals (unstable oxygen molecules that damage other molecules). In the future, whenever cells are unable to use available fuel, laboratory-produced ketones might fill the gap. Veech believes that ketone bodies could help treat neurological diseases like Alzheimer's, some heart conditions, and problems related to insulin deficiency or resistance. (He cautions, however, that low-carb diets, which stimulate ketosis or a high level of ketones in the bloodstream, may be dangerous for people with preexisting heart disease.)

Ketones have already proved successful in the treatment of epilepsy. Since the 1920s, severely epileptic children have been given lots of fat and not much protein or carbohydrates, a diet that induces ketosis and inhibits their seizures. The small percentage of children who do not respond to current drugs are still fed fat-laden meals based on butter and cream. Fasting has also been used to treat epilepsy. In 1921, eighteen epileptic patients improved after three weeks of fasting.

In Matthew 17, when Jesus was asked how he had cured a boy possessed of demons or seizures, he said, "This kind does not leave but by prayer and fasting."

Extreme ketosis—too many acids circulating in the bloodstream—is ketoacidosis, which occurs in diabetes and in an absence of insulin. The lack of insulin causes fatty acids to pour unchecked out of fatty tissues, along with a dangerous rise in glucose. High levels of glucose dehydrate the body, and a cascade of events can end in a diabetic coma or death.

In the milder ketosis caused by fasting, insulin levels are low but present, keeping fatty acids under control. Low insulin levels help move glucose into only the most important glucose-dependent cells. The blood sugar level drops in the first three to five days of fasting, rises slightly, and then stays constant. Excess ketones are secreted in the urine and released through the respiratory system in what fasters call "acetone breath."

The brain can increase its use of ketone bodies until they account for two-thirds of its energy use. The liver and kidneys now need to produce less glucose from amino acids. The body uses its resources more judiciously, too. After a week of fasting, the surface areas of the intestinal walls are greatly reduced. A shrinking gut frees energy normally required for the maintenance of the stomach and small intestine. Other systems start getting less attention—the skin perhaps, and hair. Proponents of fasting believe that the body starts consuming its abnormal cells, its arterial plaque, and the odd tumor. Anything that can be spared is converted into something useful. The body is adjusting, readjusting, fine-tuning its response to disaster. The body is designed to eat the world; now it must eat itself.

It's a kind of miracle.

. . .

Not eating seems to be innately religious. Physical hunger is too good a metaphor for spiritual hunger, and to fast is to proclaim your hunger for what is not physical—for the divine. At the same time, physical hunger is a metaphor for the desires of the body, and to fast is to overcome those desires, to trade the body for the spirit. All the major religions expect their followers to fast in some way, at some time, and for the same reasons: to focus the mind on God, to control the body, to prepare for revelation, and to offer penance or sacrifice.

Siddhartha Gautama was a child of wealthy parents who left his luxuriant home in search of Enlightenment, some peace at the

heart of the world's pain. First the future Buddha tried yogic discipline, a mental practice designed to take him outside normal consciousness. Although he succeeded in reaching a trancelike state of
non-self, he returned always to his old self, the push-pull of desire
and fear. Next the future Buddha tried asceticism, the denial of the
body's needs. For six years, he ran through the forest naked and
hungry. His hair fell out. His teeth loosened. His skin hung in folds.
Sculptures of the fasting Buddha show a skeletal figure, the ribs
protruding like a musical instrument. Again Gautama was successful, this time in becoming a great ascetic. But again what he tried
to push away returned, his hunger made even more powerful. Finally
the future Buddha abandoned starvation, sat under a tree, achieved
Enlightenment, and announced the four noble truths. Life is
suffering. The cause of suffering is desire or attachment. Non-
attachment is possible. The Middle Way—shunning the extremes
of asceticism and indulgence—is the path to non-attachment.

The Buddha rejected hunger as a means to inner peace, but
the religion that bears his name does not. All the main branches
of Buddhism fast as part of their spiritual practice. Buddhist
monks and nuns often eat only one meal a day. Theravadin Buddhists fast as a way of clearing the mind. Tibetan Buddhists fast
as an aid in yogic feats, such as generating heat. Many Buddhists
fast on the Full Moon and holidays.

Hindus also fast during festivals and on the New Moon. They
may eat nothing or only eliminate certain foods. (Fasting usually
means no food, or no food and water, but it can be any form of
abstinence.) They fast to concentrate on the spirit. They fast to
appease their gods. In Tamil families, women fast to avert the
death of their husbands or to safeguard a brother's health. Hin-
duism highlights the physical benefits of fasting, believing that it

rests the digestive system, clears the body of toxins, and leads to greater health.

Moslems do not eat or drink from sunrise to sunset during the month of Ramadan, as well as on twenty other occasions. They fast because the Qur'an said, "Fasting is ordained for you as it was ordained for those before you." They fast in repentance and in celebration. During Ramadan, Moslems acknowledge food as a gift from God. After a day of denial, the evening meal is meant to be enjoyed.

Jews fast from sundown to sundown on Yom Kipper, the Day of Atonement. They fast on other days to facilitate *teshuva*, or a return to God. They fast out of a sense of history, to commemorate the destruction of a temple or the invasion of an army. They fast in respect for the suffering of their ancestors. They fast for special favors or to produce a trancelike state. The Torah says that soldiers in a Jewish army should spend a day fasting before they go to war. Then they will know that their success comes from God, not from their own strength.

In a Taoist story, from the master Chuang Tzu, a woodworker produced a bell stand so beautiful it seemed to be the work of spirits. When questioned, the woodworker responded:

When I am going to make a bell stand, I never let it wear out my energy. I always fast in order to still my mind. When I have fasted for three days, I no longer have any thought of congratulations or rewards, of titles or stipends. When I have fasted for five days, I no longer have any thought of praise or blame, of skill or clumsiness. And when I have fasted for seven days, I am so still that I forget I have four limbs and a form and body. By that time, the ruler and his court no longer exist for me. My skill is concentrated and all outside distractions fade away. After that I go into the mountain forest and examine the Heavenly nature of the trees. If I find one of superlative form, and I can see a bell stand there, I put my hand to the job of carving; if not, I let it go. This way I am simply matching up Heaven with Heaven.

Mormons fast the first Sunday of each month. One version is to skip two meals; another is to forsake food and water for twenty-four hours. They may give the money they save by not eating to charity. They may fast as a petition. They may fast for advice.

Catholics fast on Ash Wednesday and on all Fridays during Lent, usually by eating only one meal. They fast to control their fleshly desires. They fast to do penance for their sins. They fast in solidarity with the poor.

In tribal religions across the world, fasting promotes spiritual visions or dreams. Fasting may be related to rituals of mourning or initiation or magic. For the Plains Indians of North America, fasting could help a warrior gain supernatural powers. Native Americans still fast during ceremonies and in conjunction with the sweat lodge. They fast in thanksgiving or for a gift from the Creator. "One can go into the hills," Long Standing Bear Chief, a contemporary Blackfoot, says, "or even fast and seek a vision in your back yard."

. . .

Today, Protestant and Evangelical churches are in a renaissance of fasting. Some leaders go without food for forty days in imitation of Christ in the desert. They fast for revival. They fast for the glory of God. They cite the New Testament in which the followers of John the Baptist—a man who fasted often on honey and locusts—go to Jesus and ask why His disciples do not fast too. Jesus replied, "Can the children of the bride chamber fast while the bridegroom is with them? As long as they have the bridegroom with them, they cannot fast. But the days will come, when the bridegroom shall be taken away from them, and then shall they fast in those days."

This is exactly what happened. After the crucifixion of Christ, in the first and second centuries, ascetic movements in Christianity were popular. Church authorities warned against excess, but excessive fasting was not uncommon, especially among the desert fathers, men and women who retreated into barren lands and lived as hermits or in cloistered groups. For other Christians, the rituals of fasting on certain days brought them together as a community and prepared the way for the greater feast, the corporate act of receiving the body and blood of Christ.

In the fourth century, the Greek writer we call pseudo-Athanasius wrote: "Observe what fasting does: it heals disease, dries up the bodily humors, casts out demons, chases away wicked thoughts, makes the mind clearer and the heart pure, sanctifies the body and places the person before the throne of God."

The author, who was writing a tract on female virginity, believed that virgins were especially well served by fasting. Saint Jerome, an important scholar of the time, went so far as to say that the preservation of chastity required fasting. Alternately, a full stomach excited the body and genitals. For men, too, especially monks, fasting was the answer to sexual dreams and nocturnal emissions. "For fasting is the life of the angels," pseudo-Athanasius concluded, "and the one who makes use of it has angelic rank."

How much to fast, how much God wants us to fast, has always been a dilemma. In 384 AD, Jerome wrote in praise of a twelve-year-old who "performed fasting for refreshment; hunger was her recreation." He told another young woman to let her companions be those who were "thin with fasting, of pallid countenance." Such a pale, thin girl could expect to be the Bride of Christ, and "When sleep comes upon you, He will come behind the wall and He will put His hand through the opening and will touch your body. You will rise, trembling, and say: 'I languish with love.'"

Later, Roman society would be scandalized when a widow under Jerome's influence pursued asceticism too vigorously. At her death, the accusations burst forth: the girl had been killed by overzealous fasting and the monks responsible should be driven from the city. Now Jerome would begin to warn more prudently against long fasts that lasted for weeks and omitted all food.

For these Christians, the link between food and spirituality was not simple: all of the body was linked to all of the soul. As the philosopher John Cassian wrote in the fifth century, "With any change of eating, the quality of our purity is necessarily changed as well." Along with combating sexual desire, fasting also put the sword to gluttony, which some Christians of that day counted as the first major vice, with gluttony leading to lust, and lust to avarice, and down the line to anger, vainglory, and pride. Gluttony was especially stubborn, for the body needs food to eat. Sexual desire was almost as bad since we need sex for procreation. For such physical sins, a physical cure.

By the thirteenth century, and for the next four hundred years, fasting had become a female specialty. Catherine of Siena ate only herbs, a handful a day. Clare of Assisi ate nothing on Mondays, Wednesday, and Fridays. Saint Veronica often fasted for three days at a time; on Fridays she permitted herself five orange seeds in honor of the five wounds of Christ. Many women became famous for surviving on nothing but the Holy Host for years. By fasting, women ate the food that was God, they literally fed from God, and they deepened their role as the Bride of Christ. By fasting, they became a channel through which they could serve others. Women saints were said to multiply crumbs into loaves, exude oil from their breasts, and cure disease with their saliva. Like Christ, the faster suffered, and through her suffering tasted His essence. For these women, fasting and food were part of a symbolic language, a lived metaphor expressed in the body.

Like any language, fasting was open to miscommunication. Even the saints worried that their aversion to food came from the devil, not God. When she was twenty-six years old, Catherine of Siena wrote to church authorities: "I am sure you have no other motive than the desire to honor God and care for my health, fearing a demonic siege and self-deception. About this fear, Father, particularly about the matter of eating, I am not surprised; I assure you not only you are fearful, I myself tremble with fear of a demonic trick." Fasting could be seen as female willfulness, a rebellion against families who wanted their daughters to marry, bear children, and live a conventional life. Fasting was sometimes forbidden by one's own confessor. Catherine of Siena eventually died of self-starvation; throughout her short life, her fasting was an offering received by her church with ambivalence.

With the decline of medieval culture, religious fasting also declined. There were still cases of "miraculous maids" who lived without food, often young girls from poor families. But now they had to be investigated, their claims verified. In 1546, the mother of a fraudulent fasting maid in Germany was tortured, garroted, and burned, her daughter branded and imprisoned for life. In 1600, however, the fourteen-year-old daughter of an English locksmith was deemed truly miraculous because of the lack of ex-crement: "her privy parts were cleaned thence nothing fell to ground." The young woman's emaciation was also obvious, her belly lean and dried as befitted someone who had "neither eate or drinke" for almost three years.

The appearance of fasting girls continued into the eighteenth and nineteenth centuries. For some of these, fasting only meant juice diets or very small amounts of food. At the same time, new medical theories began to emerge, alternate ideas as to how a woman's inner "fermentation" or ovarian activity could allow her to live without food, how she might even get substance from elements in the air.

In 1807, an Englishwoman with two illegitimate children stopped eating. Soon she was a celebrity, investigated by the Royal College of Physicians. For five years, Ann Moore and her village were financially rewarded, in small part, from tourists, doctors, and religious seekers. Eventually, Ann agreed to be put under a watch by local authorities. Within a week, she was near death. Now her daughter confessed to feeding her mother through bits of food wrapped in a handkerchief or transferred through kisses. Ann Moore, who had admittedly survived on very little nourishment for a long time, agreed to having "occasionally taken sustenance for the last six years." Her name became synonymous with deceit, an ignominious end to the miraculous maid.

The tradition, of course, did not really end. In Portugal, Alessandrina Maria del Costa was bedridden and paralyzed by the age of twenty-one. For over thirteen years, she was alleged to live entirely on the Eucharist, neither eating nor drinking, sub-jected to many medical exams. She died in 1955. Therese Neu-mann was a German who displayed the stigmata. Except for one consecrated wafer a day, she was said to have fasted, for thirty-nine years until her death in 1962.

For other Christians, the extremes of self-mortification and the scandals of the nineteenth century tainted fasting as a spiritual exercise. In the 1980s, when Quaker theologian Richard Foster researched Christian fasting, he was unable to find a single book published on the subject from 1861 to 1954. Foster wrote his own book that revived fasting as a form of worship. "Fasting," Richard Foster wrote, "can bring breakthroughs in the spiritual realm that will never happen in any other way. It is a means of God's grace and blessing that should not be neglected any longer."

Fasting has returned to the Christian world, and any major bookstore can provide a dozen titles for inspiration. In *A Hunger for God*, Baptist minister John Piper defined New Testament fasting as different from the mourning and petitions of the Old Testament. The Christian faster is yearning for the Second Coming of the bridegroom. His faith is a joyful homesickness, a "hunger for all the fullness of God." Moreover, "the greatest enemy of hunger for God is not poison but apple pie. It is not the banquet of the wicked that dulls our appetite for heaven, but endless nibbling at the table of the world." For Piper, fasting could be a modest withdrawal from the table of the world, a respite from our "prime-time dribble of triviality" and from all the pleasures that in our desire for them become substitutes for God.

In *The Fasting Key*, evangelist Mark Nysewander said that fasting opens the door to healing, holiness, protection from disasters, revelation, and more. The author admitted, "I don't like to fast. I don't feel good when I fast. I get headaches. Many times I feel weak, jumpy, and depressed. But that is God's way of showing me who I really am." The faster sees his dependency on God, and the revelation is physical. "When I empty myself of food, I not only know I am weak, I experience it."

In America, organizations like the U.S. Prayer Track, World Vision, Campus Crusade for Christ, and the National Association of Evangelicals have hosted hugely successful group fasts. In 2000, a movement known as The Call attracted 400,000 people to Washington, D.C., for a day of fasting and prayer. Similar mass events followed in New York and Texas, each one a direct response to Joel 2 in the Bible: "Declare a holy fast . . . call a sacred assembly . . . bring together the elders, gather the children."

John Piper also points to South Korea, where he says 30 percent of the population are evangelicals and where fasting has become commonplace. In South Korea's missionary churches, over twenty thousand people say they have completed a forty-day fast.

The new spiritual fasting can claim material rewards. Jerry Falwell, chancellor of Liberty University, went on two forty-day fasts during a time when his university was in financial crisis. He lost eighty-two pounds and the university received fifty million dollars in donations. For some supporters, a fast gets you God's attention and then gets you what you want, a remission of cancer or a new job. Recently, The Call urged its followers to "be the hinge of history" as they fasted to reverse the court case that removed prayer from public schools.

In traditional Christianity, there is another role for fasting. From Isaiah 58, "Is not this the fast I have chosen? To loose the bands of wickedness, to undo the heavy burdens, and to let the oppressed go free, and that ye break every yoke? Is it not to deal thy bread to the hungry, and that thou bring the poor that are cast out to thy house?"

"Fasting," John Piper wrote, "is meant to awaken us to the hunger of the world, not just our own hunger." The annual thirty-hour fasts promoted by World Vision raise millions of dollars for famine relief and food aid. "Break my heart," prayed the founder of those fasts, "with the things that break the heart of God."

. . .

My own fast was secular. It was the miracle of ketosis that interested me, the magic of ketone bodies. Doctors who recommend fasts also recommend that they be done under medical supervision. I agree more completely now than I did before. At the time, I was cocky: *Hey, I'm fifty years old. I think I know what I'm doing.* I was in good health, and I had a physician friend I could call for advice. Of course, I read some books on how to fast, although I didn't read them carefully enough.

Hunger was not the problem. Commonly, skipping the first few meals is the hardest. The stomach rumbles and tut-tuts. The stomach is belligerent. By the third day, however, hunger is more like a computer program that keeps coming up on screen. You feel a slight headache, and the program pops up: go into the kitchen. All I had to do was click the "x" box. In general, people who stop eating suffer less from hunger than those who eat less. In a complete fast, the shrinking and unused gut probably stops producing and sending hunger hormones. The brain becomes confused. The metabolism of fasting turns off a few switches. Ketosis feeds the body now, which forgets its other life.

The problem was boredom. As the novelty of not-eating wore off, the boredom of not eating loomed large. We stitch the day together with flavors and rewards, the gold star of chocolate, lunch with a friend. Not eating made me see that more clearly. On the second night, too, fifty-four hours without food, I woke up, went to check on my teenage son, and fell down three times. These were blackouts, slamming hard on a tile floor, a kind of death or extinction. I staggered up, took a few steps, and fell down again. Finally back in bed, I knew what I had done wrong. Dimly now, I remembered reading about this.

In *Fasting and Eating for Health*, Dr. Joel Fuhrman warned that due to lowered blood pressure, especially falling blood pressure on standing up, "the chief risk or side effect of fasting is the chance of fainting and injury in the fall." Dr. Fuhrman was careful to instruct his patients to lie down whenever they felt light-headed and to never jump out of bed in the middle of the night.

On the third day of my fast, I was bruised and chastened, with a bump on my forehead. I called my physician friend and had my blood pressure checked. By this time, it was slightly high. My pulse was very high. The body has two main responses to low blood pressure: increase heart rate or constrict blood vessels. My heart was beating faster to compensate.

I understood one thing now about hunger. It makes people fall down. Hunger makes people lose consciousness, wake dazed, scrabble on the floor, feel extinguished, feel like a bug. Fasting lowers blood pressure for a number of reasons. An initial loss of salts and water and the breakdown of fat tissue into fatty acids is mildly dehydrating. This lowers blood volume, which means lower blood pressure. In prolonged fasting, the thyroid produces fewer hormones, slowing down the body's metabolism and conserving energy; this also results in low blood pressure. Weight loss lowers blood pressure too. In addition, Joel Fuhrman believes that fasting reduces the underlying cause of high blood pressure by removing fatty, hardened plaque in the blood vessels.

On the fourth day, I stayed in bed. I smelled like paint thinner. I was cold. I wanted a hot bath, but the books said I shouldn't. Extremes of temperature use up too much energy. I brooded on this. I second-guessed my life. We make choices at a time when they are all possibility, air and flight. Years later, we find ourselves exploring the walls surrounding us, the hardened shape of choice.

People who fast seven days and more often say how happy they are. They feel special, like a miracle maid. All those ketones dancing in their brain make them see things differently. They smell better and hear better. They feel light. For moments at a time, they forget they have four limbs, a form, and a body. The ruler and his court no longer exist for them. Their skill is concentrated. They examine the heavenly nature of trees. They sit in their backyard staring up at a maple leaf, matching Heaven with Heaven.

I didn't experience that, although I think I would have if I had continued past the fourth day. I have tried to be honest about why I did not. I didn't want food anymore. I wanted the meaning behind food. I wanted to go for a walk. I wanted to clean the house. I wanted the Middle Way. I wanted to be the panther "leaping around the cage whose noble body, furnished almost to the bursting point with all that it needed, seemed to carry freedom around with it too." I didn't like the perspective of someone who had to be careful when she stood up. I was bored. So I ate an orange.

THIRTY DAYS

IN 1848, SEVENTEEN-YEAR-OLD HENRY S. TANNER immigrated to the United States from England and became a carriage maker. Five years later, he and his new wife were students at the Eclectic Medicine School in Cincinnati, Ohio, where they were taught the then–scientifically correct opinion that human beings could not survive more than ten days without food. Dr. Tanner got into the business of electrothermal baths and explored the effects of fasting and food on health. He began with week-long fasts and the theory that carrots made a person nervous, turnips sweet-tempered, and french beans irritable. Some of his ideas were self-fulfilling. According to one newspaper account, when he insisted that his wife eat three pounds of french beans a day, she pelted him with crockery and later sued for divorce. By 1877, Henry was single, middle-aged, rheumatic, asthmatic, and depressed. He decided to commit suicide by not eating past the proverbial ten days. "Life to me under the circumstances was not worth living," he later wrote. "I had found a shortcut and had made up my mind to rest from physical suffering in the arms of death." Ten days passed, and Henry Tanner felt rcmarkably well. Under a doctor's supervision, he continued fasting for thirty-one more days. His asthma, rheumatism, and chronic pain disappeared. Both physicians were amazed.

On June 28, 1880, Henry Tanner began a forty-day fast at Clarendon Hall in New York City. In part, he was responding to the controversy over an American fasting maid who had demonstrated psychic powers as a result of having not eaten for the last fourteen years. Prominent doctors pooh-poohed the woman and challenged her to their version of a duel: a forty-day around-the-clock watch by members of the New York Neurological Society. In that time, she could neither eat nor drink. The psychic refused out of modesty, unwilling to be inspected by male physicians. Tanner gallantly agreed to take her place. He would show the unbelievers that fasting was not only natural, but healthy. He would prove to these materialists the power of the human will, that there "is something beside oxygen, hydrogen, and carbon in the brain."

By the eleventh day of the performance, hundreds of visitors were paying twenty-five cents to see the dehydrated Dr. Tanner, who mostly sat doing nothing, occasionally applying wet cloths to his head or reading through a pile of letters. Eventually, he resumed taking water but continued to abstain from food. By the twenty-eighth day, a museum had offered to stuff his body should he die, and the newspapers were following the story as a "wrestling match with the invisible fiend of hunger," as well as a "starvation comedy." On the fortieth day, having lost thirty-five pounds, the doctor broke his fast before an audience of thousands. No one was too surprised when he ate a peach and drank a glass of rice milk. But some gasped as he went on to devour a watermelon, followed in the next few hours by a broiled beefsteak and a half-pound of sirloin. Always a short, stout man, he quickly gained back twenty pounds, survived his indiscriminate refeeding, and took to the lecture circuit promoting his ideas of the "recuperative power of the self."

The scientific world was unmoved. Respectable physicians called the experiment humbug, and the *New York Times* referred to it as Tanner's folly. They were both wrong. The ability of humans to live without food for weeks and even months would soon be proved in carefully controlled experiments in the best laboratories. The theory of fasting for health, called therapeutic fasting, would also become widely popular.

Then there was competitive fasting. In Madison Square Garden, an athlete who had fasted seven days lifted a half-ton of weights more than a thousand times in less than thirty-six minutes. Hunger artists, like the one in Franz Kafka's story, amused crowds in the capitals of Europe. Usually men took up this challenge, although a few women competed too, like Clare De Serval, the "Apostle of Hunger," who fasted publicly in 1910 in a glass box. Mostly these displays were about money and entertainment, similar to the "living skeletons" that could still be found in carnivals and freak shows.

In 1912, a team of scientists at the Carnegie Nutrition Laboratory in Boston began the first scientific study of a thirty-day fast, using as their subject Mr. A. Levanzin, a man from Malta. The agreement between them covered Levanzin's traveling expenses, with a bonus if the experiment was successful.

A. Levanzin was forty years old, five foot six inches tall, and under 150 pounds at the beginning of the fast. He had some legal training, some medical background, and a lively career as a political writer and publisher. In a journal written in the nutrition laboratory, he remembered his first experience in therapeutic fasting, "About two and a half years ago, while I was over-eating, obese, neurasthenic, pessimistic, and with a shattered nervous system, I chanced to read in the *Contemporary Review* an article about fasting. It was a flash of light that struck me vividly." Both Levanzin and his wife realized they had discovered "the right path to health and happiness." They read everything they could find on the subject, in several languages, and took a year to prepare for their first lengthy fast. Mrs. Levanzin, who had suffered from indigestion and insomnia, broke hers on the thirty-third day and her husband on the fortieth. Throughout this time, they felt fine, and their ailments disappeared.

Later, Levanzin fasted for twelve days to ward off cholera and claimed to have cured his daughter of smallpox by having her fast for seventeen days. At the Carnegie Nutrition Laboratory, the authors of the final 250-page report "A Study in Prolonged Fasting," published in 1915, described their subject as "a propagandist with pronounced views on all subjects." His personality was contentious, his flesh soft and flabby, his habits sedentary. His familiarity with the literature on fasting both astounded and irritated the scientists. Concerning the experiment, he made numerous helpful suggestions they did not appreciate. He was also unwilling to do certain tests. He refused to exercise daily on the ergometer, for example, "declaring that he never rode the bicycle and thought it beneath his dignity and that although the bicycle was used in Malta, it had not been used by his people."

During the thirty days, Levanzin lived in the laboratory. Occasionally, he was taken out for car rides or up to the roof for fresh air. Although difficult at times, he was dedicated to the project,

and the researchers felt certain that he drank nothing but dis-
tilled water and would refuse any offer of food. In their opinion,
Levanzin was "that type of man who can narrow his horizon about
an idea and stubbornly resist all invasions." After the first week,
his observers found him to be frequently depressed and sometimes irritable. In his journal, he complained that the monotony
of the program was the hardest to bear. His mental acuity never
seemed to diminish. Throughout the fast, he was always ready to
discuss subjects such as the Esperanto language, the politics of
Malta, and theories of mental telepathy and spiritualism. On the
fifteenth day, Levanzin went for a carriage ride in which another
passenger noted, "He talked very excitedly during the hour of the
drive; in fact, he talked continuously."

Physically, the pasty coating on Levanzin's tongue grew more
pronounced, until the ninth day, when it began to lessen. Certain
reflexes—the jump of his knee—disappeared. As more weeks
passed, his muscle strength declined and his eyesight improved.
He lost twenty eight pounds and his body looked emaciated.

On the thirty-first day, the end of the fast, Levanzin wrote, "I
am feeling very well, very uplifted, and I wished to prolong it further, at least to forty days because I do not feel yet any trace of
hunger at all. . . . During the fast I did not feel the least uncomfortable sensation except the bad taste of my coated tongue, and
the catarrh and congestion of my eyes that I had at the start have
nearly disappeared."

The refeeding did not go as well. The subject suffered from
constipation and vomiting and seemed to his doctors to be utterly
wretched and discouraged. At one point, Levanzin accused the
researchers of trying to poison him. On the fourth day after taking food, "he was very emotional, his voice scarcely audible. He

wept as he talked. His hands trembled and his face was bathed in perspiration." Suspicious and resentful at having to break the fast "early," he left the lab to recuperate in a nearby hospital.

The study's conclusions were unremarkable. The subject ended thirty days of fasting without any permanent damage or change to his physical or mental health.

A few years later, researcher Howard Marsh wrote of his experience going twelve days without food:

> Heart pounds greatly and more or less constantly, particularly at the pit of the stomach; also beats rapidly and flutters at stair-climbing. Unable to do work afternoon or evening. Great lassitude and discomfort of general nature and in head. Throat dry but no desire for water or liking of it. Pains in head, eyes, back, legs, especially knees and calves—lying, sitting or standing. No nausea but sense of instability in the stomach—of being easily upset. Feelings of sympathy, joy, reverence, etc. all are reduced in quality—lifeless in fact.

The researcher's colleague, his wife, was also fasting. In her description, the bath gave no pleasure, she felt like crying during the mental tests, and she was startled by sudden noises. She experienced little hunger, although at night she dreamed of food, "fried cucumbers and chopped olives being used as padding around some mechanical apparatus." Everything tired her and she couldn't "speed up beyond a jog trot."

These researchers noted a fall in their body temperature, a weakened respiratory system, and a decrease in their white blood cell count. Their mouths were dry, their saliva bitter. Unlike Levanzin, they felt fatigued and without vitality.

Through the rest of the twentieth century, a pattern emerged. Scientists were happy to document the consequences of fasting: what happened in the blood, in the brain, in the liver. But from their first reaction to Henry Tanner's performance, they seemed disinclined to explore any possible benefit. The idea of not eating was counterintuitive. Fasting was early associated with spiritualism and psychic powers and later with an alternative medicine lacking the rigor of Western science. Fasting was also a non-consumptive therapy that did not lead to the creation of any new drug or product.

There were exceptions. Studies in 1910 and 1915 looked at therapeutic fasting for diabetes. French neurologists suggested fasting for epileptics. In the 1960s, doctors explored fasting as the answer to obesity.

A paper published in 1964 in *The Journal of the American Medical Association* discussed eleven patients who had fasted for 12 to 117 days. Patients "who had much to gain by attaining a normal weight" tolerated the fast better and longer. Hunger was experienced for the first two to four days but was surprisingly mild in all cases. Patients became less thirsty and drank less. Physical strength and energy slowly declined, although the younger patients up to forty-five years remained moderately active. One-third became sensitive to cold. Blood pressure dropped for everyone. For three patients, the fast was terminated because of extremely low blood pressure. Two patients developed gout and had to resume feeding. For most subjects, blood levels of glucose, fatty acids, amino acids, and electrolytes remained in the normal range. Three patients had very low levels of glucose, but no resulting symptoms. Two of the patients were diabetic, but required no medication during the fast. Only one patient showed signs of vitamin deficiency after two months without food. Her bleeding gums and skin problems quickly resolved with a supplement. Four patients developed mild anemia. The weight loss ranged from eighteen pounds on the twelve-day fast to 116 pounds on the 117-day fast. "The most astonishing aspect of this study," the paper concluded, "to the patient and to the physician, was the ease with which prolonged starvation was tolerated."

In 1966, another study published in the reputable British journal *The Lancet* fasted thirteen patients, ages seventeen to seventy-one. A fifty-four-year-old woman, weighing 262 pounds, fasted for 249 days. She experienced recurrent edema (water retained in tissues, often causing swollen hands or feet), but otherwise remained healthy, losing seventy-four pounds. By the end of the fast, her arthritic knee was no longer painful. A thirty-year-old woman, weighing 281 pounds, fasted for 236 days and lost ninety-seven pounds. All of her blood tests remained normal, as did her menstrual periods. Another seventy-one-year-old woman fasted for fifty days and suffered only from a dry mouth. All the patients spoke of their increased well-being and, in some cases, "frank euphoria."

In 1973, a Scottish journal published the successful fast of Mr. A. B. for 382 days. The study also noted five patients who had died during other experiments in prolonged fasting: two from heart failure, one from a small-bowel obstruction, and two during the refeeding phase. In the end, considering these risks, fasting was abandoned as a cure for obesity.

Since then, research on fasting has been relatively scanty. In the 1970s, the Japanese looked at fasting for psychosomatic diseases, such as depression, anxiety, and neurosis. The Scandinavians considered fasting in the treatment of rheumatoid arthritis.

In the 1980s, fasting seemed successful for eighty-eight Americans with a mild to moderate infection of the pancreas. A seven- to ten-day fast gave relief to Taiwanese workers poisoned with PCBs. Other studies have connected fasting with the successful treatment of protozoan parasites, duodenal ulcers, high blood pressure, and diabetes.

Outside the hospitals and laboratories, outside the academic committees who determine funding, therapeutic fasting has continued to thrive, modestly, in its own parallel world. Founded in 1948, the National Health Association emphasizes the body's natural self-healing abilities. A parallel British society dates from 1956. In Europe, especially in Germany, fasting cures and spas did a brisk business up through the 1960s. By the mid-1970s, an infusion of Eastern culture into the West had brought ideas of "cleansing the body" through fasting, which became an established practice in alternative medicine. Today, the International Association of Hygienic Physicians supports professionals who specialize in therapeutic fasting. In this world, fasting is effective against a range of problems, from asthma to uterine fibroids. Most of the proof is anecdotal.

In this world, fasting helps the body detoxify. In every one of our cells, wastes are produced as a natural part of metabolism. Free radicals are one example of cellular waste. We also take in toxins like chemicals, pesticides, and bacteria. Normally, we break down toxins in the liver and excrete them through the kidneys, as well as through our skin and mucous membranes. Hygienic physicians believe that a high-fat, high-protein diet stresses our natural ability to detoxify and that periodic fasts may be necessary to clean out the system. Toxins that have been stored or deposited in fat and other tissues are released and can now be eliminated. A body without food also begins to break down superfluous tissues besides fat—abnormal cells, tumors, arterial plaque.

In this world, fasting allows the digestion system to "rest." The immune system also "rests," no longer having to deal with food allergies and ingested toxins. Fasting lowers blood pressure and glucose levels, which can be good. (High blood pressure damages the circulatory system. A consistently high level of glucose can also damage tissues, especially blood vessels.) Medical doctors, like Joel Fuhrman, note that fasting thins the blood and aids in the breakdown of blood clots. Ketosis decreases free radical damage and may have other positive effects at the level of the cell membrane and microcirculation. By using up fat, fasting reduces leptin levels, which regulate the inflammatory and immune response. In mice that model human multiple sclerosis, high levels of leptin are associated with symptoms of the disease. A very low level in starved or leptin-deficient mice inhibits these symptoms. All this may be why people with digestive disorders, food allergies, diabetes, heart problems, and autoimmune diseases seem to get better when they fast.

In this world, it is important to remember that there are two stages to not eating. The fasting stage is as long as the body can support itself without harm on stored reserves in the tissues, whether that be three days or twelve days or thirty days or more. Eating less food, as in a juice fast, does not have the same effect as not eating any food. If the diet includes a supply of carbohydrates, ketosis will not take place, and the body will continue to use fats, carbohydrates, and proteins in much the same way. Also, hunger will be experienced differently than in a complete fast. Hormonal levels will be different.

⟳ The second stage of not eating is starvation, which begins when the stored reserves are used up or have dropped dangerously low. Semi-starvation or malnutrition is the result of insufficient food or the wrong kind of food or both. Fasting for health does not mean starving for health.

Some people should not fast. A rare inborn error of metabolism may mean that their body cannot easily break down glycogen or that they incompletely break down fatty acids or that they cannot convert the ammonia produced from protein breakdown into urea. Instead of miraculously living on air and sunshine, they go into a coma.

Eating is the corollary to fasting. Natural hygienic physicians have very definite ideas about what people should eat and should not eat in order to maintain the benefits of a fast. Read their books. You already know what they are going to say.

. . .

North of San Francisco, California, between the Pacific Ocean and the vineyards of Napa Valley, the TrueNorth Health Center is surrounded by rolling hills and landscaped gardens. Alan Goldhamer, a doctor of chiropractic medicine, opened the center in 1984 as a place where patients could take supervised, prolonged fasts. Alan had just finished an internship at a fasting center in Australia where he found himself saying, over and over, "If *this* patient gets well, I'll really be convinced." His patients kept getting well, and today TrueNorth is a twenty-bed facility with a staff of nine that includes a medical doctor and clinical psychologist. Here, Alan has overseen more than 5,000 fasts for people with chronic and acute disease. At TrueNorth, staff members have also been caught muttering to themselves, "If *this* patient gets well, I'll really be convinced." They all arrive at the same place.

Alan Goldhamer believes that humans are motivated by the instincts that motivate all animals: seek pleasure, avoid pain, conserve energy. In the past, that triad was an internal compass pointing in the direction he calls TrueNorth. The compass told us where to go and what to do for health and happiness. In terms of diet, modern humans are now being misdirected, overwhelmed, and seduced by "pleasure traps" that appeal to our hard-wired excitement in finding a high-energy, high-caloric food source. The concentrated pleasure of chocolate cake creates an intense eating experience to which we gratefully become addicted.

"For our ancestors, the path toward more pleasure, with less pain, and for less effort was always the right path to choose," Alan says. "Unfortunately, this is no longer the case." TrueNorth has shifted. Alan makes a nice distinction between pleasure, a response of the nervous system to a specific stimulus, and happiness, an extended mood that occurs when we perceive the balance of our experiences to be positive. Happiness is created by the ongoing act of making progress toward our goals. The goal at TrueNorth is health.

Alan believes that therapeutic fasting is adaptive—like ketosis and like our ability to store fat. The ability of the body to heal itself through fasting is something we share with animals that rest and stop eating when they are sick or injured. Their lack of appetite is part of their cure. "When an unhealthy animal fasts," Alan says, "it is fighting for its life." That, more or less, is what you go to TrueNorth to do: to retreat like an animal from the clamor of the world, to hide in your nest of leaves and grass, to rest and dream and eat nothing as you wait for your body to heal.

Sometimes you give your fur or genitals a few licks. Sometimes you drag yourself outside to drink from a puddle of water. Sometimes you drowse in the sun.

Actually, at TrueNorth, you share a nicely decorated, semi-private room for $109 per day or ask for a private room at a higher cost. The bedspreads are cheerful, as in any good hotel, and a print of flowers hangs on the wall. The first thing you will do is have a physical exam. After that, your blood pressure and pulse will be checked daily, and you will have weekly blood and urine tests. You will not be given vitamin and mineral supplements. Most natural hygienic physicians believe that even in a long fast you get enough vitamins from the breakdown of body tissues. Also, your need for micronutrients is reduced as your metabolism slows down. You will not be given an enema. You will drink lots of distilled water. In the morning, you will be visited by one of the doctors of chiropractic medicine, and you will go to a short educational program. You will be encouraged to sunbathe for ten to twenty minutes a day, perhaps lounging on the patio or going for a slow walk in the garden. Chiropractic treatments are available at a modest cost. So is psychotherapy.

You must stay on the premises. You will be urged, even required, to rest. Muscular activity increases the body's need for glucose, a need now being supplied by the conversion of protein, as well as the glycerol in fat. You are free to read or work on a computer or listen to music (using earphones) or sit in the TV room. In the evening, you will be visited again by one of the staff. Any medication will be given and supervised by the staff. You may not smoke or drink alcohol or take non-prescription drugs or wear perfume or use nail polish or spray anything from an aerosol can. You should bring casual, layered clothing, including a robe and slippers.

Refeeding is crucial. After a fast, you must stay for no less than half the length of the time you fasted. A fourteen-day fast is a twenty-one-day stay. Refeeding begins with juices, then raw food, then the addition of cooked vegetables.

Most people agree that fasting makes healthy food taste good, a reset on your taste buds, and TrueNorth has a chef who serves fresh fruit and steamed vegetables just as you would expect them to be served in northern California. A carrot is extraordinarily sweet, unsalted broccoli rich and flavorful. A fast-food cheese-burger, on the other hand, would smell of chemicals. Fasting is an interlude, a big Cyclone fence between you and your former self. Alan says, "In my clinical experience, I have seen nothing that re-motely approaches the effectiveness of water-only fasting to en-courage the adoption of a healthy diet. Not the fear of excruciating pain, not the fear of a lifetime of obesity. Not even the fear of death itself."

In a study directed by Alan, 90 percent of 174 patients with hypertension who fasted at TrueNorth got their blood pressure down to normal without the use of drugs. Patients who stayed on a low-salt, low-fat, plant-based diet were able to keep their blood pressure down, also without the use of drugs. Fasting, Alan be-lieves, was "a happiness strategy" to break a metabolic cycle and the habits that perpetuated it.

It is not a vacation. Or maybe it is a bad vacation, with not much to do and unexpected discomforts. These can include headaches, hunger, heartburn, insomnia, dizziness, nausea, feel-ings of cold, coated tongue, body odor, aching limbs, palpitations, fatigue, mucous discharge, and visual and hearing disturbances. "It's not fun," Alan says blandly. "It can be an intense and some-times unpleasant experience."

The following symptoms might cause a doctor to break a patient's fast: a sudden drop in blood pressure, delirium, prolonged hypothermia, a rapid or slow or irregular pulse, extreme weakness, renal insufficiency, extreme vomiting or diarrhea, gastrointestinal bleeding, gout, heart arrhythmia, or emotional distress. These things are rare. But they happen.

Who should not fast? "Contraindications are few," Alan says, mentioning pregnancy, certain cancers, and diseases related to metabolism. Mainly, though, people should not fast if they are afraid to fast.

In fasting literature, stories take the place of clinical trials. Sarah says that fasting saved her life. Gabriel became fertile. Barbara walks easily now. Carlos is a new man. If you are like me, you are glad for these people but not convinced. Still, consider this: in March 2001, the International Union of Operating Engineers included water-fasting as a fully covered medical benefit for all of its members and spouses with high blood pressure or diabetes. Over 400,000 strong, these guys are heavy equipment operators, mechanics, and surveyors. The IUOE also represents nurses and some health workers. They are the kind of people with a bottom line: does it work?

. . .

You haven't eaten for thirty days. Mostly you stay in bed, huddling for warmth under the purple-and-green cover. Every day, tiny bits of your body are being converted into the grams of glucose your brain and other tissues still need. Your electrolytes—potassium, sodium, and chlorides—are stable. Your cholesterol and triglyceride levels are high, since your body is running on fat. Your glucose and blood pressure levels are low. You are very careful when you stand up. You move slowly. Time moves slowly. You have lost thirty-two pounds, and your face is drawn. You try to drink as much water as you can, although you don't really like water anymore. You just want to lie here and read or lie here and not read. You don't sleep well at night. Instead, you think about when you can eat again. This is desire, not hunger. Everyone around you is very kind.

. . .

If the benefits of fasting for health are controversial, the benefits of eating less are not. Mice given less food but all their essential nutrients age more slowly and live longer than mice on a normal diet. Mice programmed genetically to develop Alzheimer's or Parkinson's disease develop the disease more slowly on a calorie-restricted diet. Calorie-restricted mice perform better at memory tasks and learning than other mice. Calorie restriction also inhibits the growth of cancerous tumors in mice genetically designed to have cancer. It is not just about mice, either. Every animal on a calorie-restricted diet, from Labrador retrievers to rhesus monkeys, has gained in some way.

In an experiment begun by the National Institute on Aging in 1987, one group of rhesus monkeys, of all ages, was fed normally, while another group was given 30 percent less food. Twice the monkeys eating more food have died, and twice as many have problems with cancer, heart disease, diabetes, and failing kidneys. Scientists are cautious about how these studies relate to people. Human trials have been hard to organize for the obvious reason: researchers can't find enough volunteers.

Serendipitously, in 1991 four men and four women sealed themselves up for two years in a project called Biosphere II, a domed space of three acres open to sunlight and electrical power and closed, otherwise, to the outside world. Here they grew their own food and maintained a self-sustained ecological system. When some crops failed, the Biospherians had to reduce their calories to 1,784 a day for six months. Gradually that number rose to two thousand a day for the remaining eighteen months. The diet was high in nutrients, but low in fat and animal protein. Since all the crew worked an eighty-hour week, with lots of physical labor, this amounted to a restricted diet. The men lost 19 percent of their body weight and the women 13 percent. Their blood pressure; their white blood cell count; their levels of glucose, insulin, and cholesterol declined. They hardly ever got sick. They had plenty of energy.

The results from Biosphere II parallel the animal studies. Other reports from the Biosphere confirm something else: people on a calorie-restricted diet get hungry, maybe a little cranky, maybe a little controlling. At each meal, the eight men and women in their brave new world watched each other carefully. No one wanted anyone else to get more than a fair share. On their part, the calorie-restricted monkeys in the National Institute on Aging study get more excited at dinnertime than the monkeys in the control group.

Some hunger, apparently, is good for you. But almost any hunger triggers a negative emotional response. The mechanisms of hunger are a bit of a tease.

We don't really know why calorie restriction would make us healthier or live longer. In a few years, new studies funded by the National Institute of Aging may answer some of our questions.

We do know that consistent high levels of glucose and insulin cause aging-like damage, as does high blood pressure. We know that metabolization, the breakdown of food and the creation of energy in a cell, generates free radicals or unstable oxygen molecules that damage other molecules. Part of aging is the accumulation of these damaged bits of matter. Calorie restriction decreases this oxidative stress. Calorie restriction slows metabolism, lowers body temperature, and results in weight loss. Calorie restriction may cause changes in genes that turn off or on during the normal aging process.

Then there is *hormesis*: the beneficial actions resulting from the response of an organism to low-intensity stress. *Hormesis* helps an animal deal better with sudden high-intensity stress, such as wounds, high or low temperatures, or toxins. Calorie-restricted mice also respond better to these things. A calorie-restricted diet is a kind of stress that puts us in survival mode, which might then evoke responses that benefit us.

Intermittent fasting may kick in the same defenses as calorie restriction. During another experiment, lab workers got tired of going in to feed the mice every Saturday and Sunday, so they started leaving enough food for two days and skipping a day. They noticed that the mice that ate all their food and then fasted had drops in cholesterol and blood pressure and lived longer. Further studies showed that alternate-day fasting in mice resulted in even greater health benefits than calorie restriction. The National Institute on Aging has begun to advertise for volunteers for a fasting experiment in older people.

. . .

By and large, the medical world remains dubious. Fasting for health does not have support from the American Medical Association. Psychologists also warn that a lifestyle that promotes fasting can trigger or exacerbate an eating disorder. At the same time, the placebo effect, the power of suggestion and of the mind, is something that Western medicine has come to recognize. If people feel better, it's hard to argue.

By and large, the fasting world still relies on stories. Sarah and Gabriel and Barbara and Carlos do feel better, and they are too impatient for the scientific method, which requires you to doubt your own theory and then spend years trying to disprove it.

Into this space, this unbridged gap, the International Union of Operating Engineers takes the leap.

THE
HUNGER STRIKE

HUNGER IS A FORM OF COMMUNICATION. WHEN we fast for health, we are having a conversation with the body. When we fast as a Jew or Catholic, Moslem or Hindu, we are having a conversation with God. These are private discussions and often silent. Hunger strikes are different. Almost always, they are loud and public, like a messy family argument the whole neighborhood can hear. The man or woman fasting for change wants the world to know and judge. To know and act. The conversation is with the world. Hunger is a demand, a cry, and if that cry is ignored, hunger will only call out more urgently, seeking its audience until they also begin to call and cry and demand, and there are many voices now, and hunger has become theatre—a tragedy, perhaps, or a farce. In a hunger strike, the end is not yet written. The play unfolds.

Hunger strikers believe that the voice of hunger has a power disproportionate to its source. Hunger can strengthen the weak, inspire the timid, bully the powerful. The voice of hunger can free the oppressed and right injustice. It can alter history. In the story of David and Goliath, hunger is David's stone. Thousands of lives will change because of one man's hunger. And this is true. This has happened.

. . .

Fasting as protest is not new. In medieval Ireland, fasting against a person was part of the legal system. If a man felt you had wronged him and died hungry on your doorstep, you became responsible for his debts. In ancient India, "sitting dharna" was also a fast to the death to protest injury or injustice. Both countries have produced the most influential hunger strikes of the twentieth century. A bit oddly, the twentieth century can be called the heyday of hunger strikes. This renaissance is due partly to the media, the way a newspaper and now the Internet can publicize drama. We may as well have a more modern way of seeing hunger, as an anomaly rather than the normal human condition, an affront to our ideas of who we are.

The English suffragettes are credited with reviving the hunger strike. They already had a flair for theatre. In January 1909, a member of the Women's Freedom League shouted down at the House of Commons from a dirigible balloon emblazoned with the slogan "Votes for Women," while dozens of league members were being arrested below. Accompanied by a befuddled delivery boy, suffragettes would often send themselves as human letters to the prime minister. Dressed in prison clothes, they also liked to jump out of fake prison vans to chalk up the sidewalk. Sometimes drama won over common sense. Thrown in jail, Lady Constance Lytton thought it might be a good idea to carve the words "Votes for Women" onto her chest.

For the suffragettes, jail was desirable. Sylvia Pankhurst, a leader in the militant suffragette movement, described a scene that took place with her mother, Mrs. Pankhurst, who stoutly refused to leave the entrance to the House of Commons. As a police officer pushed the elder woman away, she lightly tapped him on the cheek. "I know why you did that," the man said. "Must I do it again?" Mrs. Pankhurst asked quietly. Yes, she must if she wanted to be arrested, and so she did, and so she was. Meanwhile that very afternoon, the activists began a new policy of breaking government windows. Not wanting to hurt anyone inside, they wrapped the stones in paper, tied them with string, broke the glass, and neatly dropped the missile in the hole. Window breakers were at once taken away by the authorities. "It was a pitiable sight," the *Daily Telegraph* reported, "the earnest faces of these frail, high-spirited young women roughly handled by the worried police."

By now, another strategy had begun to prove itself. After one woman, who Sylvia Pankhurst remembered as "neither young nor strong but possessed . . . of a cheerful courage," was arrested for graffiti, she demanded to be treated as a political prisoner and declared she would not eat until that time. The Governor assured her there would be no concession and she would be left to die. Meanwhile, she was offered tempting food such as fish, bananas, and milk. After ninety-one hours, the suffragette was set free. In her history of the movement, Sylvia Pankhurst wrote, "Her release was received with great rejoicing and intense relief by the few who were aware of her ordeal. She had staked her life on the reluctance of the government to let a woman die and had won the test—a brave deed. Her leap in the dark led to freedom. Dozens of women were ready to follow, believing the way had been found to the vote itself."

The authorities understood this threat and responded accordingly. Fasting suffragettes in jail were now treated roughly and put into punishment cells, the rooms cold, the floors damp. Sometimes their injuries were ignored. As they continued to fast, delicacies like jam and chicken and fruit were again left in their cells. (Sylvia Pankhurst, like many fasters, felt little hunger. Although the colors of the food pleased her in the drab surroundings, she had no more "desire to eat the still life groups on my table than if they had been a painting or a vase of flowers.") The women often fainted. They had stomach cramps. Their hearts beat erratically. After some time had passed, no matter what their sentence, they were released. Some had fasted for as little as three days, some for six, one woman for thirty. In every case, the suffragettes were right in their appraisal of the government: there was a reluctance to let a woman die. It was matched only by the reluctance to let a woman vote.

Through the summer of 1909, the suffragettes continued their campaign of throwing stones and heckling politicians. Mrs. Pankhurst was even accused of inciting the bombing of the chancellor of the exchequer's house; she pleaded not guilty. Now when the prisoners began their hunger strikes, the government was in no mood to release them. Instead, the women were force-fed with a rubber tube through the nose or mouth. The method was harsh. Some of the women suffered nervous breakdowns or had serious and long-lasting physical injuries. Over a hundred physicians signed a letter addressed to the prime minister against force-feeding. One doctor declared in a London newspaper, "As a medical man without any particular feeling for the cause of the suffragettes, I consider forcible feeding by the method employed an act of brutality beyond common endurance."

Years later, Sylvia Pankhurst remembered her first experience with the horror of a woman who had been raped. That evening, at the appointed time, she knew "they were coming" and she waited in her cell frightened and outraged. In a clothes basket, she gathered together what she could find to throw at her attackers: a cup, a plate, her shoes. She heard their footsteps. Then six wardresses burst into the room, and Sylvia could not use her "missiles" against women she saw as tools and victims. Instead she struggled as they threw her down and pinned her on the bed. She closed her eyes and clenched her teeth. Suddenly a man's hands tried to force open her mouth. A steel instrument bit against her gums, searching for a gap. She jerked her head away, breathing faster and faster, trying to scream. There was "a stab of sharp, intolerable agony." Something gradually pried her jaws apart, "the pain was like having teeth drawn," and she felt the tube being shoved down into her stomach. After a few minutes, it was withdrawn. She promptly vomited, and they left her on the bed, sobbing.

So it went, day after day. Her gums were continually bleeding, her mouth bruised and swollen. Sometimes she fainted during the procedure. Afterward, her whole body ached. "Infinitely worse than the pain was the sense of degradation: the very fight that one made against the outrage was shattering one's nerves and self-control." Sometimes during the struggle, she experienced a sense of "many selves," one aloof and calm, another ruthless and unswerving, and "Sometimes, breaking forth, it seemed, from the inner depths of my being, came outraged, violated, tortured selves; waves of emotion, fear, indignation, wildly up surging." Alone in her cell, the prisoner grew to fear that these emotions would overwhelm her.

Seriously ill, Sylvia Pankhurst was finally set free and allowed to recover. Another suffragette almost died when a feeding tube entered the trachea and food poured into her lungs. Soon after, in the spring of 1911, the English parliament passed the Cat and Mouse Act, which allowed authorities to release prisoners while they were on hunger strike and take them back later to serve their sentences. As a determined "mouse," Sylvia Pankhurst would go in and out of prison many times, sometimes refusing water as well as food, sometimes walking incessantly, refusing to sleep or rest.

In 1913, the House of Commons again debated the problem of hunger strikers. Various ideas were considered. Perhaps the suffragettes could be deported? Or sent to an island prison? Or placed in a lunatic asylum? None of it seemed quite feasible. Perhaps, one lord suggested, if a few died of hunger, the rest would be cowed. But as another man complained, "So far from putting an end to militancy, I believe it would be the greatest incentive to militancy which could ever happen." On this point, the suffragettes and the lords agreed. Sylvia Pankhurst wrote, "Comradeship in sacrifice is a thing of power able to lift its members to the high peaks of transcendent being." For every woman who died, others would come forward for the honor of martyrdom.

A year later, World War I interrupted the momentum of the suffragettes, most of whom began to work for the war effort instead. In 1918, British women finally won partial voting rights and in 1928 the same rights as men. American suffragettes also fought for the vote, went to prison, refused to eat, and got their privileges in 1920.

In Ireland, nationalists who opposed the British occupation of their country had begun to use the hunger strike as well. In 1917, a nationalist died in prison after being force-fed. Forty thousand people followed his funeral procession through the streets of Dublin. In 1920, the lord mayor of Cork died of a hunger strike after seventy-four days without food. His words became a touchstone for future strikers, "It is not those who inflict the most but those who will suffer the most who will conquer."

. . .

As Sylvia Pankhurst waited in her jail cell for the wardresses to come, she prepared to fight, arming herself with a cup, a plate, and her shoes. Meanwhile, Mohandas Gandhi was a lawyer in British-controlled South Africa, fighting non-violently for the rights of Indian subjects. The hunger strike was not yet part of his politics of civil disobedience. But Gandhi's mother had been a religious Hindi who fasted throughout his childhood, on religious holidays and as personal atonement, and her son naturally followed that discipline. He saw eating much as he saw sex, something to be tolerated for the sake of survival and reproduction, but also a sensual pleasure to resist—a distraction from the greater intimacy with God. Gandhi came to believe strongly in the health benefits of fasting and would advise readers through an article in *Young India* to fast "(1) if you are constipated, (2) if you are anemic, (3) if you are feverish, (4) if you have indigestion, (5) if you have a headache, (6) if you are rheumatic, (7) if you are gouty, (8) if you are fretting and foaming, (9) if you are depressed, (10) if you are overjoyed."

In 1913, Gandhi and his family were living in South Africa in an ashram where he served as a leader and teacher. During one of his trips away, two boys at the ashram suffered a "moral fall."

There is no record of what that fall was. In his autobiography, Gandhi wrote only that "the news came upon me like a thunderbolt" and he rushed home. During that journey, his duty became clear. Gandhi felt that any teacher was partially responsible for the lapse of a pupil and so a penance was required of him. Only then would the boys understand the seriousness of their transgression. He imposed on himself a fast for seven days, followed by one meal a day for four and a half months. Immediately, he felt greatly relieved: "The anger against the guilty parties subsided and gave place to the purest pity for them."

In Gandhi's account, his fast pained everybody but cleared the air. The bond between him and the children under his care became stronger and truer. This fast was not for health, and it was not for religious reasons. It was a dialogue with the world, in this case, the small world of the ashram. Importantly, "Where there is no true love between the teacher and the pupil, where the pupil's delinquency has not touched the very being of the teacher and where the pupil has no respect for the teacher, fasting is out of place and may even be harmful."

In 1914, after twenty years as a political and social activist in South Africa, Gandhi returned to India as an international hero. In 1918, he was asked to help textile workers in the industrial city of Ahmedabad fight for better pay. He advised the workers to go on a labor strike with the pledge that, no matter how long the strike lasted, they would never resort to violence, begging, or dishonest work. The first two weeks went well. The workers showed courage and self-restraint and came in the thousands to shout their pledge at mass meetings. The mill owners, however, refused to bargain—despite their friendliness and goodwill toward Gandhi. Increasingly, the workers grew discouraged and aggressive, and Gandhi feared "an outbreak of rowdyism." Finally, at one meeting, "Unbidden and all by themselves the words came to my lips." Gandhi declared to the laborers that he would not eat until they had fulfilled their pledge, either reaching a peaceful settlement or leaving the mills altogether.

Gandhi's first public hunger strike, at the age of forty-eight, was not against the mill owners, but against the mill workers, his own people. For Gandhi, the flaw in this plan was that the mill owners might also feel pressured by the fast and be coerced into an agreement. Instead, Gandhi wanted them to resolve the conflict because they saw the justness of the strikers' cause, because the action of the strike was nonviolent, and because they were moved by an inner and lasting transformation. Earnestly, he begged them not to let his fast affect their position.

The mill owners saw it differently. Gandhi was revered as a national saint, a Mahatma or Great Soul. Various female relatives of the owners had already become greatly attached to him. The workers' demands were met three days later.

"I fasted to reform those who loved me," Gandhi would one day tell his friend Louis Fisher. "You cannot fast against a tyrant." Nor could you fast for personal gain. "I can fast against my father to cure him of a vice, but I may not in order to get his inheritance."

For the next thirty years, Mahatma Gandhi worked for India's independence from England. But he rarely fasted against the British. His strategy remained that of civil disobedience, and for these actions he was often arrested and jailed. He became more concerned with how India achieved her freedom than with when. If a campaign turned violent, if his followers could not hold to his high ideals, he saw that as defeat. Increasingly, too, the violence that depressed him most was not between the Indians and Britons, but between the Moslems and Hindus, and between the Hindus and their own Untouchables—a subgroup of the caste system.

In 1924, Mahatma Gandhi went on a twenty-one-day fast for Hindu-Moslem friendship. He chose to fast in the house of a Moslem leader. After twelve days, he wrote that the struggle was no longer for "a change of heart among Englishmen" but for a change of heart among Hindus and Moslems. Before they could think of freedom, they had to be "brave enough to love one another" and to tolerate each other's religion. "This requires faith in oneself. And faith in oneself is faith in God. If we have that faith, we shall cease to fear one another."

In 1932, Indian and British leaders began working on a form of Indian self-government. Gandhi declared a fast to the death when the British suggested a constitution that would establish three separate electorates for Moslems, Hindus, and Untouchables. Gandhi believed that to give the Untouchables a separate electorate would divide them further from their fellow Hindus and undo what work had been done to get rid of the caste system. The British quickly demurred to whatever the Hindus and Untouchables decided. Gandhi said his fast was "intended to sting Hindu consciousness into right religious action." The man who represented the Untouchables, however, called the fast a political stunt.

Gandhi was now sixty-two years old and in a British jail. Early on, this fast badly affected him. He drank little water and seemed listless. He could not stand nor walk, but had to be carried to his bath on a stretcher. He complained of sharp pains, and his blood pressure rose alarmingly high.

The news media in India followed every detail. Those who could read told the story to those who could not, and they told others. All over the country, Hindus prayed for their beloved

Great Soul. His desire had been to make each one of them feel responsible for his life, and they seemed to understand. From the first day of the fast, Hindu temples that had previously denied entrance to Untouchables opened their doors. Hindu schoolchildren sat next to Untouchables during class. Untouchables could now use wells and roads once forbidden. Thousands of well-known Hindus let it be known that they had personally taken food from the hand of an Untouchable. Villages, towns, cities, organizations, associations, and unions passed resolutions banning prejudice.

Louis Fisher wrote, "The fast could not kill the curse of untouchability which was more than three thousand years old. Access to a temple is not access to a job. . . . But after the fast, untouchability forfeited its public approval; the belief in it was destroyed." To practice untouchability now was to be branded a bigot or a reactionary. Gandhi's fast "snapped a long chain that stretched back into antiquity and had enslaved tens of millions. Some links of the chain remained. . . . But nobody would forge new links; nobody would link the links together again."

By the fifth day of the fast, Gandhi seemed near death. He whispered to his wife who should inherit his few personal belongings. By now, Hindu and Untouchable leaders had worked out an agreement, but nothing could be official until the British government consented as well. The new pact was telegraphed to London on a Sunday. Ministers left their homes, hurried to Downing Street, poured over the documents, and telegraphed back their approval early Monday morning. That afternoon, Gandhi accepted a glass of orange juice.

Eight months later, still in jail, he went on a twenty-one-day fast for his own purification and for the purification of his ashram, where a pretty American woman had caused another moral fall. The British government felt sure their prisoner would die in this longer fast and immediately released him. But Gandhi fasted easily now, with few problems.

In another three months, he launched another campaign of civil disobedience, was arrested again, and sentenced to another year in prison. This time, Gandhi did fast in protest of the British authorities. When he declined in health, he was again unconditionally released. In 1935, he fasted seven days in penance when a Gandhi supporter struck an anti-Untouchable with a stick. In 1939, he went on a "fast to the death" against a Moslem Raj for the civil liberties of the people of Rajkot. At the age of sixty-nine, he showed symptoms of heart disease now and fasts were becoming more dangerous.

In 1942, in jail again for civil disobedience, Gandhi went on a twenty-one-day fast to protest the continual imprisonment of activists like himself. In a letter to the viceroy, he wrote, "Usually during my fasts I take water with the addition of salts. But nowadays my system refuses water. This time therefore I propose to add juices of citrus fruit to make water drinkable. For my wish is not to fast unto death, but to survive the ordeal, if God wills." Gandhi hinted that he would end the fast if the government responded appropriately. The viceroy wrote back saying that he regarded the fast as a form of blackmail and reminded Gandhi that he had once said he would only fast against those who loved him. Later, reminiscent of the earlier Cat and Mouse Act, the government offered to release the activist while he fasted. Gandhi replied that if he were released, he would have no need to fast. At that, the government said he could invite into jail as many doctors

as he wished. On the thirteenth day, Gandhi was badly nauseated, his kidneys failing, his pulse feeble, and his skin cold. A few
drops of fruit juice seemed to help, and he survived to the end of
the twenty-one days.

In 1947, India achieved full independence. The cost was parti-
tion. Within India, Moslem leaders insisted they be able to form
the separate state of Pakistan. Gandhi opposed this division but
came to see it as necessary. Over twelve million people began to
move, Hindus and Sikhs fleeing the new Pakistan and Moslems
fleeing a volatile India. In a series of murders and massacres, half a
million people died—burned or stabbed or shot or dismembered.
In Calcutta, 23 percent of the population remained Moslem and
the city suffered religious riots for over a year. Gandhi came to
town as the guest of a Moslem householder and declared he would
begin a fast "to end only if and when sanity returns to Calcutta."
Three days later, police officers could report that there had been no
sign of violence for twenty-four hours. Hindu, Moslem, and Christian leaders, merchants and workers, pledged to keep the peace.
The Great Soul had a glass of sweet lime juice, and Calcutta remained free of bloodshed for months to come.

From Calcutta, Gandhi went to Delhi, where his presence also
calmed the city. The worst of the violence stopped, but the Mahatma was not satisfied. Once more, "in a flash," the idea came to
him. He would fast to the death, a fast directed to the conscience
of all: Hindu and Moslem, the new citizens of India, and the new
citizens of Pakistan. He would break his fast only when Delhi,
India's capital, knew real peace. According to Louis Fisher, he declared to one congregation, "I have not the slightest desire that
the fast should be ended as soon as possible. It matters little if

the ecstatic wishes of a fool like me are realized and the fast is never broken. I am content to wait as long as it is necessary."

Gandhi was seventy-eight years old. This would be his last hunger strike. As before, water nauseated him. Again, his kidneys began to fail, and he lost weight rapidly. By the third day, he was 107 pounds, his blood pressure at 140/98. Half asleep or half-conscious, he lay curled on a cot, his head and body covered by a white cloth while lines of people moved slowly past, ten feet away, weeping and praying. At his request, the Indian government hurried to pay the newly created Pakistan 180 million dollars, its share of India's assets. Committees met to design a pledge that would satisfy the Mahatma, one to be signed by the major leaders of India, from the president of the Indian Congress to the Chief of Police in Delhi. The pledge bound these men to protect the life, property, and faith of Moslems; to support annual Moslem festivals; to ensure that Moslems could move freely in Delhi and elsewhere; and to return to Moslems those mosques that had been overtaken by Hindus and Sikhs. Everyone knew Gandhi would not give in easily. In a written statement, he warned that India would not be served if its politicians misled him with the idea of saving his life: "They should know that I never feel so happy as when I am fasting for the spirit. This fast has brought me higher hitherto. No one need disturb this happy state unless he can honestly claim that in his journey he has turned deliberately from Satan toward God."

On the sixth day, Gandhi wept when he spoke to the men offering their pledge. His great desire was to go to Pakistan and plead for peace there. But how could he know that he was not being deceived now? Leaders from both religions stepped forward to reassure him. Slowly, Gandhi drank a glass of orange juice.

Twelve days later, he was assassinated by a Hindu who opposed his vision of tolerance and religious diversity.

. . .

Altogether, Mahatma Gandhi underwent seventeen public hunger strikes and uncounted personal ones. (He once fasted against a married Indian woman who had seduced his twenty-year-old son. The woman was persuaded to cut her hair in remorse, and his son would not be allowed to marry for another fifteen years.) Gandhi had nine rules for fasting: (1) Conserve your energy, both physical and mental, from the very beginning; (2) Cease to think of food while you are fasting; (3) Drink as much cold water as you can; (4) Have a warm sponge bath daily; (5) Take an enema regularly; (6) Sleep as much as possible in the open air; (7) Bathe in the morning air; (8) Think of anything else but your fast; and (9) No matter from what motive you are fasting, during this precious time think of your Maker and of your reliance on Him and His other creations and you will make discoveries you may not have dreamed of.

Occasionally, the Mahatma broke his own rules, especially the first one: conserve your energy, both physical and mental. Those fasts in which he felt the most urgency, the greatest need for a successful outcome, were the ones that threatened his life the most. Desire and fear—these have their metabolic costs.

Gandhi's endurance in fasting was also limited by his size and weight. He never went over twenty-one days and probably could not have survived for much longer. During the first days of fasting, ketone bodies are produced more quickly in lean subjects than in the obese. After a week, there are other differences, with important disadvantages among the lean. Obese fasters not only have more fat to burn; they also have more body protein and fat-free tissue, and they use these resources at a slower rate. In part, this may be because glucose is now being produced from two sources—protein and the glycerol in fat. The obese have more fat and thus more glycerol. Moreover, the obese become better adapted to the use of ketone bodies and so need less glucose. In one study of a prolonged fast, the breakdown of fat into ketones provided 94 percent of the energy needs of obese subjects compared to only 78 percent in lean subjects.

· · ·

By the last half of the twentieth century, hunger strikes had become relatively common. One historian documented over two hundred in fifty-two countries between 1972 and 1982. In this time, twenty-three hunger strikers died.

Ten of those deaths were Irish Republicans imprisoned by the British outside Belfast. Very little about this hunger strike was Gandhian. All the fasters were associated with the Irish Republican Army, which pursued terrorism as a means to the end of British control over Northern Ireland. Most of the prisoners had possessed illegal weapons. One of them, Francis Hughes, admitted to setting bombs and shooting people. Their demand was a familiar one, to be treated as political prisoners rather than criminals. This was not a fast to reform those you love and who love you. This was a hunger strike based on hate and the will to defeat a hated enemy. The Irish Republicans saw the British as conquerors. "Foremost in my mind," wrote Bobby Sands, the first Irish Republican Army prisoner to die, "is the thought that there can never be peace in Ireland until the foreign, oppressive British presence is removed, leaving all the Irish people as a unit to control their own affairs, free in mind and body." The British, notably then–Prime Minister Margaret Thatcher, saw the Irish Republican Army as murderers who targeted innocent men, women, and children. Neither side felt it could morally retreat from its position. The deaths of the hunger strikers seemed almost inevitable, a kind of blood sacrifice.

Doctors often see the turning point in a hunger strike after forty days. Pain and illness begin to dominate. The body does not have enough energy to do the basic tasks of cellular function: to move material across membranes, to synthesize molecules, to break up molecules, to create new cells. The body is extracting vitamins and protein from unnecessary tissue and these include the muscles in the eyes. First you have double vision. Then your sight dims. You vomit green bile. Your speech is slurred. You can't hear very well. You have jaundice. You have scurvy from lack of Vitamin C. Your gums begin to bleed. You may be bleeding into your stomach and intestines. You may have thiamine deficiency, which weakens the muscles of the heart and causes lesions in the central and peripheral nervous system. As your nerve fibers degenerate, you feel a sharp pain down your arms. One day, you cannot move your legs. Niacin deficiency may be the reason for the sores in your mouth. You may have what is called "skin breakdown." This is the process of starving to death. All the things you lack—vitamins, minerals, glucose, renal function, hope—work synergistically. Your body is falling apart in so many ways and in so many places; you can't track a dissolution that is everywhere.

According to the 1995 *Assistance in Hunger Strikes: a Manual for Physicians and Other Health Personnel Dealing with Hunger*

Strikers, hunger strikers usually experience little mental deterioration except for apathy and some problems in concentration. The psyche "remains clear" until the final stage, which is characterized by euphoria and "global confusion," followed by a coma. Brain damage may now be irreversible, "One should not think there is time left to negotiate," the manual warns.

Twenty-seven-year-old Bobby Sands died on his sixty-sixth day of refusing food. Seven days later, Francis Hughes died on his fifty-ninth day. In eleven days, Raymond McCreesh and Patsy O'Hara both died on their sixty-first day. Two strikers lasted until their seventy-first and seventy-third day. As each man neared the end, he faced—if he were conscious—an impossible choice: going off the strike to save his life would be to deny the sacrifice of the man who had died before him. As one reporter wrote, "The validity of each death depended upon its being followed by another, the solidarity that counted was with those who had died rather than with the living." This went beyond political ideas. This was personal loyalty. Meanwhile, as each prisoner starved to death, another man took his place on the strike, so that there were always ten hungry men, so that the strike could last indefinitely.

The Belfast hunger strikes ended when the families, the mothers and sisters and fathers, rebelled against their death-watch and began to intervene. After six men had died, Paddy Quinn's mother was the first to save her son. Having fasted for thirty days, Paddy found it difficult to walk. He was so nauseated that he couldn't keep down water. He heard a constant buzzing and mumbled to himself. On his forty-seventh day, he began to have convulsions. According to journalist David Beresford, Paddy's screams of pain and delirium rang throughout the hospital corridor, so that the mothers of other hunger strikers had to cover their ears. The widow Mrs. Quinn asked the prison doctor what her son's chances would be if she did something right now. Fifty-fifty was good enough for her.

Later, the Quinn family issued a statement emphasizing "that had Paddy remained conscious we could not have taken the decision to give him medical treatment. He was determined to go on to the end." After Paddy's mother took the right of decision-making for herself, four more men died without intervention and four families stepped in to prevent their sons' death. By then, it was clear that the hunger strike was over. The prisoners ended the protest without being granted their demands, although the English government would accede to most of these within a year, quietly and voluntarily.

The courage of the ten Irish prisoners who died in the spring and summer of 1981 moved people all over the world. Many saw their refusal of food as selfless. The Catholic Church decided it was not suicide. During the eight months of the strike, violence between the factions in Ireland escalated; thirty-four civilians and thirty soldiers and police officers were killed by bombs or guns. In the end, the martyrdom of the strikers empowered the Irish Republican Army, which had previously declined in popular support. The organization decided to assassinate Margaret Thatcher. Three years later, the bomb meant for her killed five people and seriously injured thirty others.

The ethics of a hunger strike are still evolving. In Morocco, two prisoners protesting inadequate medical treatment were kept sedated and force-fed from 1985 to 1991. In Spain, the head of a hospital nutrition unit decided as "a matter of conscience" to force-feed three prisoners near death from a sixty-day strike; that doctor was later murdered by the militant group to which the prisoners belonged. In 1992, the World Medical Association reaffirmed its prohibition against force-feeding, which it described as a form of torture. The British Medical Association, however, states that prison doctors have the final decision on when to intervene in a hunger strike, and American courts have ruled that prisoners may be force-fed if their hunger strike is for better living conditions or to obtain a transfer.

The World Medical Association puts a hunger strike in the context of the doctor/patient relationship. The doctor is bound to respect the patient's autonomy. A gray area remains when a striker becomes mentally incompetent or when the prisoner's family asserts its rights or when the political situation changes while the prisoner is unconscious. The association suggests that strikers fill out a statement of non-intervention expressing their wishes in all possible circumstances and that they be given a "doctor of confidence" who acts outside the state or prison system.

In his biography of Mahatma Gandhi, psychologist Erik Erikson wrote, "Fasting, we may consider in passing, is an age-old ritual act which can serve so many motivations and exigencies that it can be as corrupt as it is sublime." At the beginning of the twenty-first century, I can go to my computer, search "hunger strike," and see this ritual act in all its many forms, stronger than ever. Twenty prisoners in Turkey starve to death to protest torture in the jail system. Two men in New Jersey fast to protest their detention under the Homeland Security Act. Dick Gregory begins a forty-day fast to protest criminal action against singer Michael Jackson, accused of molesting a child. Farmers in North America stop eating to protest genetically engineered crops. Afghan refugees in Indonesia sew their lips together to protest being denied asylum in Australia.

An American woman fasts to protest federal income taxes. Thousands of Palestinian prisoners in Israel stop eating to protest the abuse of strip searches and other punishments.

Hunger strikes are about changing the world and shaming the world. Hunger strikes balance the powerless against the powerful, the one against the many. They contrast the frailty of the body with the might of authority. As the body grows weaker, the power of authority can strangely weaken too. Sometimes those who represent authority are moved by the body. Sometimes those who give authority its power are the ones who are moved and who force change. Hunger strikers strip down to nothing and transform their nakedness. Their helplessness is their offering. Their show of weakness is their strength.

THE
HUNGER DISEASE
STUDIES

DURING WORLD WAR II, THE PSYCHIATRIST
Viktor Frankl was a prisoner in Auschwitz and Dachau. He
survived the German concentration camps, although his parents,
brother, and wife did not. After the war, Dr. Frankl founded a
school of psychotherapy that focused on the existential meaning
and responsibilities of a patient's life. Dr. Frankl understood that
the reality of death—the inevitability of death—might seem to
make human life less meaningful. But in his view, the ephemeral
nature of existence and the uncertainty of the future were bal-
anced by the decisions we make today and their deliverance into
the past, where nothing is lost and everything is stored. Here, in
these "full granaries," we salvage our joys and sorrows, heroisms
and failures. "Nothing can be undone," Frankl wrote, "and nothing
can be done away with." We all die. What matters is how we lived.

. . .

In September 1939, the Polish city Warsaw surrendered to the German army. A year later, the Nazis imposed a Quarantine Area that sealed all Jewish residents into nine square miles of the city's poorest section. Tens of thousands of Jews were sent here from other countries and parts of Poland. Eventually, almost half a million people were registered in the Warsaw ghetto, an average of seven people crowded into every available room. No one could leave the ghetto without permission. No food, except allowed rations, could be brought into the ghetto. In 1941, in occupied Poland, the allowed rations were 2,613 calories a day for Germans, 699 calories for Poles, and 184 calories for Jews. With a ration card, a Jew could legally buy a piece of bread, a bowl of soup, and nothing more. For almost three years, the official Nazi policy was starvation. The German governor of the ghetto noted, "The Jews will disappear because of hunger and need, and nothing will remain of the Jewish question but a cemetery."

From 1940 to 1943, the actual calories that a man, woman, or child lived on in the Warsaw ghetto was dependent on what they could sell and buy on the black market, mainly supplied through illegal smuggling; what they could get from Jewish relief organizations, who daily ladled out free soup at about two hundred calories a serving; what they could earn working in the ghetto or commuting outside as laborers for the Germans; and what they could beg. The very poor got about eight hundred calories a day and the rest of the population about eleven hundred. The favored and wealthy might eat as much as seventeen hundred calories. For the majority, meals were confined to dark bread and potatoes, servings of thin vegetable soup, and occasional tastes of butter, sugar, lard, or oil.

People dropped dead of hunger. They died on their way to work and in front of shops. They died at home and were dumped in alleys without clothes or identification, so that family members could keep the ration cards. The smells of death, decay, and human waste pervaded the streets. The cries of children were constant. One observer wrote of the beggars who were "on the sidewalks, in the gutters, in the house yards, in every hole and crack . . . old and young, women and children, mostly children, children upon children, aged three and up to fifteen or sixteen . . . composing refrains of lamentations and songs of woe." Commonly, a man or woman committed suicide by jumping from a high apartment building. In one often-repeated story, a woman's body overturned a large cooking pot, her brains and blood mixing in the food. Hordes of children, scrambling from their holes and cracks, fought to eat the contaminated remains.

Two hospitals in Warsaw had served the Jewish population. The Czyste Hospital, outside the Quarantine Area, was eventually closed and its patients moved into buildings within the ghetto. Supplies were low and the rooms overcrowded. Moreover, hunger existed here, too. The director, Dr. Joseph Stein, wrote in 1941 that the hospital had ceased to be a hospital and was not even a poorhouse. "The food supply is strictly a fiction. . . . The patient who has no means of providing his own food becomes swollen with hunger and soon dies—unusual progress in the history of medical treatment!" On occasion, orderlies found it difficult to distribute what meals were available, a ration of about seven hundred calories a day, since they were so hungry themselves. Doctors and nurses were allowed extra rations, five hundred grams of soup and sixty grams of bread, which they began sharing with the rest of the staff.

The Berson and Bauman Children's Hospital was already in ghetto boundaries and did not have to relocate. Still, conditions were so bad that one visitor admitted, "I had the impression that it would have been more humane not to prolong the life of these poor children." Another visitor described a five-year-old boy in the entrance hall, his face, hands, and feet bloated with edema. He had come to the hospital in the last stages of life. "The child still moves his lips, he begs for some bread. I try to feed him something. . . . Alas, his throat is swollen shut, nothing passes down, too late."

At an orphanage, a doctor paused before the crib of a three-year-old: "I look at the infant curled up—it looks like a worm. No body, just a bundle of bones, one could easily count them all. Just shake it and the bundle will disintegrate. The child lies panting, like a shot down pigeon."

About seven hundred Jewish doctors were living and working in Warsaw when the Germans took over. That number declined as doctors were killed by Nazi soldiers or died of disease and starvation. Jews, in any case, were not allowed the title of physician. They were not allowed to treat Aryans. They were not really professionals. One man remembered how the Gestapo would storm through the Czyste Hospital searching for papers and books, declaring that Jews had no right to science. To assert otherwise was illegal and subversive.

So, a group of Jewish doctors started a secret medical school. Many of the teachers were well known internationally, specialists in neurology, hematology, and bacteriophages. They held classes, gave exams, and smuggled out the results to be recorded by professors on the Aryan side. Hundreds of students participated. A few survived after the war to get credit for their work and continue their education.

Others began an ambitious research project. They did not have many medical supplies. They did not have well-lighted laboratories or reliable electricity. They lived in constant fear of losing their lives and families. Some could hardly find money to pay for food on the black market. What they did have was a subject to study—hunger—long neglected for the obvious problems in finding enough volunteers and enough corpses to autopsy, problems of ethics that did not seem relevant in the Warsaw ghetto. These scientists had plenty of starving patients and plenty of dead bodies. They began planning in November 1941, reorganized the makeshift laboratories, purchased some equipment, and started work in February 1942. They looked at seventy adults at the Czyste Hospital, forty children at the Berson and Bauman Children's Hospital, and thirty private patients. They were careful to isolate what they would come to call hunger disease and not to include patients with other complications, such as tuberculosis. Since almost all their patients died, it was easy to confirm the initial diagnosis of starvation in a later autopsy.

The Judenrat was the Jewish Council created to manage the affairs of the ghetto. Dr. Israel Milejkowski, head of the Judenrat's health department, initiated the research. A dermatologist, he wrote in the short introduction to the project's final manuscript, "Hunger was the most important factor of everyday life within the walls of the ghetto. Its symptoms consisted of crowds of beggars and corpses lying on the streets. . . . Many of our physician colleagues themselves suffered from hunger. In spite of this, nobody interrupted the work and quietly, modestly, without any advertising the work was done."

Dr. Julian Fliederbaum, a specialist in endocrinology, outlined their observations of adult starvation. The first symptoms were a dry mouth, greatly increased urination, rapid weight loss, and constant craving for food. Later, in prolonged hunger, these symptoms diminished and were replaced by pervasive weakness, apathy, and feelings of cold. People tended to curl up in the fetal position until their muscles became contracted in this form. The sensation of hunger dulled, although patients still responded aggressively to the sight of food. "We observed their weakness," the doctor wrote, "their slow movements at work, their clumsy attempts to grab a piece of bread from a doctor's hand, their running which always resulted in a fall."

Edema was commonly associated with malnutrition. Edema can take many forms, as swollen watery tissue or as a collection of fluid in spaces in the body, especially around the stomach and chest and between the joints. Within a cell, inadequate nutrition depresses the pumping mechanisms, which keep excess salt and water out. In later stages of starvation, the cell deteriorates and the distinction between in and out is lost. A lack of protein in the circulating plasma may also change the osmotic pressure in capillaries, causing fluid to leak into surrounding areas. In the Warsaw patients, edema first appeared in the face, feet, and legs. The affected tissues were pale, soft, and cold. In pitting edema, pressure on the skin left an indentation or pit that filled in slowly. Patients who did not have edema were classified as the "dry" cachexia type, a more obvious emaciation. Surprisingly, the swollen edematous patient was often at greater risk.

In the first stages of hunger disease, people looked younger as their fat deposits disappeared and the skin folds became shallower. In the second and third stages, they aged rapidly, so that a young woman might have the appearance of a sixty-year-old. Their skin was pale, dry, and scaly, even if waterlogged underneath. It looked like "cigarette paper or old parchment." Often, patients also had lice, scabies, and encrusted ringworm. They were covered with brown spots that formed clusters throughout the body, a pigmentation caused by malnutrition. Sometimes the entire face turned dirty brown. Some of the victims may have remembered the cry of Jeremiah 5: "Our skin was black like an oven because of the terrible famine."

Hair growth was abnormal, perhaps due to hormonal imbalances. Patients in puberty might have luxuriant growth on their head and in the genitals, with a fine fuzz all over the body. People thirty to fifty years old lost all their hair, even in the armpits and genitals.

The base of the tongue became smooth as the papillae atrophied. Sometimes the tongue looked blistered, and people complained of a burning sensation. Their voices grew hoarse; the mucous membranes of the larynx dried out, and throat muscles weakened.

The lungs also weakened and lost their tone. People got less air and breathed more slowly. They were more susceptible to tuberculosis and respiratory problems.

Poor blood circulation and a poor immune response contributed to high rates of infection. The body could make fewer new cells to fight bacteria and disease. A low level of fat in the blood meant that antibodies were carried less efficiently.

The atrophied gut could no longer process food. Bowel movements were bulky with blood and mucus.

Dr. Fliederbaum headed the work on the metabolization of carbohydrates. He measured low levels of glucose and insulin and a poor response to glucose given orally. Blood sugar rose only slowly and slightly after injections of adrenaline and declined only slowly and slightly after injections of insulin. Although the doctor thought he saw signs of thiamine deficiency, he concluded with obvious disappointment, "To our knowledge, no therapy with a single vitamin or with a vitamin complex is able to reverse the clinical and biochemical symptom of hunger disease."

Children suffering from hunger disease were studied separately at the Berson and Bauman Children's Hospital, directed by the pediatrician Dr. Anna Braude-Heller. From a wealthy family, Dr. Braude-Heller had a vocation for poor children and had earlier organized an orphanage and tuberculosis sanatorium. She dressed perpetually in black, in mourning for a son who had died of appendicitis. One colleague described her as a "short dark-haired lady who spoke in a deep alto voice and moved with surprising agility considering her weight."

Dr. Braude-Heller found that the earliest changes in a starving child were psychological. Children stopped playing and seemed humorless and bad-tempered. Their behavior became more adult-like. Later, they simply curled up, immobile but not asleep, for they often had insomnia. Their growth was stunted. Three- or four-year-old children were no bigger than infants; nine-year-olds looked four years younger. Their skin was also pale, dry, and pigmented, with hair growth on the neck and cheeks. Edema was present in two- to five-year-olds, while "children not disfigured by edema looked like skeletons covered with skin," their muscles atrophied and contracted into the fetal position. Even children who recovered still had an abnormal duck-like walk. Like the adults, their heart rate was slow, their blood pressure was low, their body temperature was lowered. They had a tendency to develop large clots in their veins. Most characteristically, they had diarrhea, frequent and severe, sometimes for months. These children, with unrelenting diarrhea, almost always died.

The doctors saw few signs of rickets, scurvy, or other vitamin-deficient diseases, possibly because of potatoes and vegetables in the ghetto diet. There seemed to be fewer cases than usual of diseases like chicken pox, bronchial asthma, or meningitis. Problems caused by allergies, liver or gall bladder dysfunctions, and diabetes were rare. Many of these conditions seemed "cured" in patients who had been hungry for a long time. Stomach ulcers were also uncommon, although in other parts of Europe during World War II, they increased dramatically.

Before the war, Dr. Emil Apfelbaum had been a popular cardiologist. Author of the manuscript's fourth chapter on the circulatory system in hunger disease, he wrote, "Death from long-lasting hunger is like a candle burning out slowly." For the most part, the changes in the body were adaptive, a conservation that reduced the patient's existence to a minimum. But the undernourished heart was still being overworked. With respect to declining body weight, the volume of circulating blood actually increased. There was also more water in the blood released from disintegrating tissues, and the diluted blood acted inefficiently as a carrier of nutrients and oxygen. In compensation, the speed of blood moving through the system slowed and the time of circulation lengthened, which somewhat reduced the heart's load. By this stage, the low blood pressure and low level of work done by the heart had become fixed. Even after a starving man exercised, there was no change in heart rate, stroke volume, or blood pressure. Injections of stimulants like adrenaline prompted only a sluggish response.

To measure circulatory responses, Dr. Apfelbaum used a tilt table, which tilted the subject's head down, then horizontal, and then up. To measure circulation time, the researchers poked two needles into a patient's artery, one to inject dye and one to collect blood samples every two to three seconds, measuring the return of that dye. To test the heart's response to exercise, the researchers had their patients perform fifteen sit-ups. The imagination pauses over the scene. We see the dying woman on a hospital bed, probably in her own ragged clothes since the hospital could not provide new ones, trying to survive for a few more hours or days, perhaps knowing that her death was certain, that the doctors could not save her. Instead, they wanted her to do sit-ups. Instead, they took blood samples.

In the English translation of these studies, published over thirty years later, the editor, Dr. Myron Winik, acknowledged that some techniques used by the Warsaw doctors were not only uncomfortable for their patients but possibly dangerous: "However, the authors obviously felt that the potential benefits to science far outweighed the risks involved, especially under the prevailing conditions. It is hard to find fault with their position."

One more sit-up, the doctors coaxed. One more needle. And from that, they promised, might come some meaning out of this horror, something to learn and pass on. In our imagination, the woman on the hospital bed tries to understand. She might even feel reassured by this bit of meaning accomplished in fifteen sit-ups. What does it matter if she spends her last hoard of energy and lives a few minutes less? She is hungry for meaning, too.

One importance of the hunger disease project would be in what it implied about refeeding or rehabilitation. In hunger, the heart adopts new strategies. The adaptive response becomes fixed and slow to respond to a new situation. This explains why a starved man refed too rapidly can go into cardiac arrest.

Dr. Michael Szejnman was in charge of the work on blood and bone marrow. Like his colleagues, he eliminated cases where he suspected complications or accompanying disease. He only took blood from people dying of hunger, and he found in them an acute anemia, as well as a reduced white blood cell count. In some patients, bone marrow had become fibrous and inactive. In others, bone marrow that continued to produce red blood cells seemed incapable of releasing them into the bloodstream.

The doctor tried various therapies. He added chopped liver and raw animal blood to the patient's small portion of food. He gave injections of iron and then combined a therapy of liver and iron. He gave Vitamin A. He gave blood transfusions, which in one case resulted in the patient's death. Nothing worked. At the end of his chapter, Dr. Szejnman wrote, "The best results were achieved by supplying adequate nutrition and food with an appropriate caloric value. These results could be anticipated because the only rational therapy for hunger is food." That therapy, of course—four or five meals a day, as much as two or three thousand calories a day—was not available.

The well-known ophthalmologist Dr. Simon Fajgenblat was asked to join the hunger disease project after it was underway. His chapter remains our most complete study on changes in the eyes during starvation. Dr. Fajgenblat did not see any deficiency of Vitamin A, which would have resulted in night blindness and a hardening of the cornea. He noted edema of the eyelids so that the patient seemed to be perpetually squinting, as well as growths of thick long eyelashes and a faint covering of hair on the eyelid. The whites of the eyes were often blue as the vascular tissue shone through the thin, transparent sclera. In the Warsaw patients, this symptom was associated with long brittle bones and a deficiency of calcium in the blood. Even though the doctor's study group consisted of adults under thirty, the lenses of their eyes were beginning to cloud, as though they suffered from cataracts, a disease of old age. They also had low pressure in the eye, probably a defense mechanism that allowed blood to enter the retinal area in a system with overall low blood pressure. Otherwise, their eyesight was normal.

The doctor observed the "negative attitude of the patients toward ocular examinations and treatment. It made our work difficult and frustrating. In studying vision, especially visual fields, one has to rely on the goodwill and concentration of the patient."

The director of Czyste Hospital, Dr. Joseph Stein, wrote the seventh and last chapter of the manuscript on hunger disease. Dr. Stein was described by his colleagues as a gentle man who had converted to Catholicism long before the war. Like other Christianized Jews, he and his family were sent into the ghetto. Dr. Fenigstein, his assistant, was a recently married doctor in his late twenties. Henryk Fenigstein had been wounded as a Polish soldier fighting the Germans and returned to Warsaw to study surgery. Instead, he worked in the pathology department at the relocated Czyste Hospital. The two doctors performed almost five hundred autopsies on patients they determined had died of hunger disease alone. Now they could see what the others could not—that the brain weight remained the same while the heart, liver, kidney, and spleen became small and light, that the bone marrow had a jelly-like consistency, that edema was often present in the small intestine, that other intestinal changes resembled dysentery, that the skeletal muscles had severely atrophied in 61 percent of the victims. They did microscopic studies describing minute changes in bone, brain, and liver cells. They typed up case studies with sad little details, such as the sixteen-year-old girl with a "fragile build" and third-degree bed sores, her brain "soft and bloated," her liver, kidney, and spleen atrophied, her heart "smaller than the fist of the deceased."

It was Dr. Stein who gave the introductory lecture "Life and Death" for the medical school, and who spoke again on July 6, 1942, at the first official and very secret general conference on hunger disease. Dr. Israel Milejkowski chaired the session with papers read aloud by Dr. Fliederbaum and Dr. Apfelbaum. Graphs and charts showed the progress of each phase of the study. The head of the Judenrat, Adam Czerniakow, was so impressed that he agreed to buy and smuggle in additional equipment and supplies. The scientists must have been unusually lively on this day. So much good work was getting done, important work, scientific work! As Dr. Milejkowski would write, "We will later—after the catastrophe—be able to demonstrate to the world that the murderous enemy could not destroy us. . . . The result of this work will be published and I hope it will be of great interest."

Two weeks later, the Nazis began massive deportations of the Warsaw Jews. These were called resettlement programs, although the people chosen for resettlement were simply taken by train to the death camp Treblinka, herded into fake showers, and gassed. All the street children, the beggars with their skeletal limbs and thin cries, chants, and songs, went into the first group. On the second day, they took the children from the refugee shelters. When the head of the Judenrat, Adam Czerniakow, was told he needed to supply the Germans with ten thousand Jews every day for resettlement, he went into his office and took a capsule of potassium cyanide. Dr. Milejkowski was in the building at the time but could only declare his colleague dead. On July 30, the orphanages were emptied. Sometimes the groups of children, along with the very old, were not put on freight trains but simply taken to the nearby cemetery and shot.

Even so, when the Germans posted a notice that any Jew voluntarily boarding the cattle trains for Treblinka would get three kilograms of bread and one kilogram of marmalade, hundreds went to the station, despite the rumors, despite what they knew.

A few of the researchers studying hunger disease died in that first deportation. In general, however, doctors, their immediate families, and their patients were exempted, although the Czyste Hospital again had to be abandoned and its patients transferred to other buildings. The graphs and charts from the project, the reports, the data, and the rough drafts of chapters were hurriedly gathered and hidden away. Almost half the material was lost or incomplete. The research phase was clearly over. Now the doctors held furtive meetings as to how they should proceed.

At the new Czyste Hospital, doctors registered their relatives and friends as patients in order to save them. In September, Dr. Stein was told that all hospital sites had to be vacated again. This time, 90 percent of the sick or injured were to be sent to Treblinka. The doctors themselves had to choose which ones would die. Dr. Stein also had to make selections among his staff. Some doctors gave morphine to the older patients, including their own mothers and fathers. At the Berson and Bauman Children's Hospital, a physician poisoned the babies. "Just as during those two years of real work in the hospital, I had bent down over the little beds," the woman later wrote, "so now I poured this last medicine into their tiny mouths."

By the end of September, half the hospital personnel and the majority of sick had been sent to Treblinka. Some of the remaining physicians were given right-to-life cards by the Germans. A small hospital continued for the fifty thousand or so people left in the ghetto. In January 1943, the Nazis entered these rooms, shot those who could not walk, and threw the rest into trucks where they were taken away. A few patients and doctors had already hidden in prepared underground bunkers. Others committed suicide or left in the trucks or were killed at the hospital.

In April 1943, the Germans began their final liquidation of the Warsaw ghetto. About 750 Jewish men and women fought back, among them the ophthalmologist Dr. Simon Fajgenblat. Almost all the resistance fighters were killed, as well as any remaining Jew, as the ghetto was burned and razed, building by building.

. . .

Israel Milejkowski wrote his introduction to the manuscript on hunger disease in October 1942, a few months after the first deportation. He found it ironic that he did this in an abandoned building in the cemetery, "a symbol of our living and working environment." In the January deportation of 1943, he was arrested and sent to Treblinka. According to reports, he had to be dragged cursing to the freight cars.

Dr. Fliederbaum, who had done the meticulous work on the metabolism of carbohydrates, killed himself in 1943. Together with his wife and small son, he jumped off the fourth floor of his apartment building.

Dr. Anna Braude-Heller, the pediatrician, refused many opportunities to leave the ghetto and reportedly said, "I am not going. I have agreed to send out my son with his wife and child. As long as there are Jews in the Ghetto I am needed here and here I will stay." When the children's hospital was destroyed, she continued to work as a doctor for the resistance fighters. Her body was found in April 1943.

Dr. Emil Apfelbaum, the cardiologist, also survived the 1942 deportations and in January 1943 used fake identification papers to escape to the Aryan side of Warsaw where he survived until the end of the war. At that time he changed his name to Kowalski, declaring that he hated the Germans too much to bear a German name. He was able to retrieve the final manuscript of the hunger disease study, which consisted of seven chapters that had been smuggled out of the ghetto and kept by a professor at the University of Warsaw. Dr. Apfelbaum prepared the work for publication and died a year later in 1946, possibly of a heart attack. He was fifty-six years old.

Dr. Michael Szejnman, who had studied blood and bone marrow changes in hunger disease, was also able to leave the ghetto in 1943. He was soon captured by the Gestapo and killed.

The ophthalmologist Dr. Simon Fajgenblat escaped with his wife after the July 1942 deportations and hid until the 1943 uprising. Wounded in the fighting, he later died. His wife became separated from him and managed to survive until the liberation. When she learned of her husband's death, she committed suicide.

Dr. Stein also would not leave the ghetto, saying that his responsibility was to stay with the hospital. He and his family were taken to Treblinka in January 1943.

Dr. Henryk Fenigstein was sent to a succession of camps, including Auschwitz and Dachau. He was liberated by the Americans in 1945 and began to work as a doctor in a Munich hospital. Later he moved to Toronto, Canada.

The fate of these men and women was researched by Leonard Tushnet and published in his book *The Uses of Adversity*. Many other scientists, doctors, nurses, and medical students also gave their time and energy to study hunger. Most did not survive the war.

Dr. Israel Milejkowski, who helped begin the project and who had to be dragged into the freight cars, ended his introduction to the hunger disease study with this prophecy, "And you by your work could give the henchman the answer. *Non omis moriar*. I shall not wholly die."

THE MINNESOTA
EXPERIMENT

AT THE END OF WORLD WAR II, AS OCCUPIED towns were liberated and prisoners released from concentration camps, the allies faced refeeding people who had been starving for months and even years. The English officer Jack Drummond remembered a cold day in January 1945 when he met with a group of Dutch, American, and British public health advisors: "It was frightening to realize how little any of us knew about severe starvation. In our lifetime millions of our fellow men had died in terrible famines, in China, in India, in the U.S.S.R. without these tragedies having yielded more than a few grains of knowledge of how best to deal with such situations on a scientific basis."

For a long time, scientists in America had lobbied for more research in famine relief. The government was interested but preoccupied with winning the war. In 1944, a group of private citizens at the University of Minnesota's Laboratory of Physiological Hygiene began what would be called the Minnesota Experiment, the first long-term, controlled study on the effects of semi-starvation. The project was headed by Dr. Ancel Keys, director of the lab, who had just developed the K-rations for the army. Funding sources included pacifist groups like the American Society of Friends and the Brethren Service Committee. The volunteers were conscientious objectors, Quakers and Mennonites eager to participate in work that meant, according to the scientists, "a long period of discomfort, severe restriction of personal freedom, and some real hazard."

The study began in November with a three-month control period, followed by six months of semi-starvation, followed by three months of refeeding. The goal for each subject was to lose 24 percent of body weight, mimicking the weight loss seen in famine. (Autopsies done in the Warsaw ghetto showed that death from starvation involved a loss of 30 to 50 percent of body weight.) The diet was one a Warsaw Jew would recognize: brown bread, potatoes, cereals, turnips, and cabbage, with occasional tastes of meat, butter, and sugar. Nothing like this had ever been done before or would ever be done again.

"It undressed us," concluded one subject. "Those who we thought would be strong were weak; those who we surely thought would take a beating held up best. . . . I am proud of what I did. My protruding ribs were my battle scars. . . . It was something great, something incomprehensible."

The results of the Minnesota Experiment were published in 1950 in the two-volume epic *The Biology of Human Starvation*, over thirteen hundred pages long, heavy as a sack of flour. Up to the last moment, the authors included the newest research appearing in various languages. The hunger disease studies of the Warsaw ghetto, still our most detailed portrait of extreme starvation, had been published in French in 1946. Doctors at a Belgium prison and a French mental hospital had written up their observations on inmates who had their daily calories reduced to between fifteen hundred and eighteen hundred during the war. The 1941–42 Siege of Leningrad, in which the Germans successfully prevented food from entering the city for over nine months, resulted in a number of scientific papers. The report of the Dutch government on the 1944–45 famine in the Western Netherlands came out in 1948. There were monographs on refeeding from places like Dachau, and field data had been gathered from the Japanese internment camps. World War II turned out to be a cornucopia of starvation research—a wealth of hunger.

. . .

It wasn't easy being a conscientious objector during the Good War. Sixteen million Americans answered the call to defend the world against Nazism and Fascism. Forty-two thousand men decided that their religious or moral beliefs prevented them from killing another human being, under any circumstances. As one activist said after the bombing of Pearl Harbor, "Being a pacifist between wars is like being a vegetarian between meals." Six thousand conscientious objectors ended up in jail for refusing to register for the draft or cooperate with federal laws; twenty-five thousand served as non-combatants in the armed forces; and twelve thousand entered the Civilian Public Service, where they worked as laborers, fire fighters, and aides in mental hospitals. As the war continued, these conscientious objectors grew increasingly restive. In an oral history compiled later, one man complained, "My God, you're talking about planting trees and the world's on fire!" Another remembered, "This is what finally got under my skin more than anything else: the sense of not sharing the fate of one's generation but of sort of coasting alongside all of that; you couldn't feel you were part of anything terribly significant in what you were doing."

Partly out of the desire to share the fate of one's generation, conscientious objectors became medical guinea pigs. They wore lice-infested underwear in order to test insecticide sprays and powders. They were deliberately infected with typhus and malaria and pneumonia. They ingested feces as part of a hepatitis study. They were put in decompression chambers that simulated altitudes of twenty thousand feet. They lived in rooms where the temperatures dropped to below freezing, a month at twenty degrees, a month at zero degrees. They were willingly too hot, too cold, anemic, jaundiced, feverish, itchy. When Dr. Keys at the University of Minnesota sent out a recruiting pamphlet titled "Will You Starve That They Be Better Fed?" over a hundred men volunteered. About half were rejected. Thirty-six were chosen as subjects in the experiment, and another eighteen as assistants and staff.

All the men had to be in good health, physically and mentally. They had to have considerable social skills, able to get along with others in a situation that would test everyone's limits. They had to be interested in relief work and rehabilitation. The men finally selected ranged in age from twenty to thirty-three. All were white, with at least a year of college education. Eighteen already had college degrees. They had a variety of body types, and they came from a variety of economic backgrounds: rich, poor, and middle-class.

Being a guinea pig was a full-time, forty-eight-hour-a-week job. The men lived in the upper floor of the Minnesota laboratory in dormitory-style bedrooms, with a nearby lounge, library, and classrooms. They worked fifteen hours a week doing laundry or clerical work, cleaning in the lab or helping in the kitchen. They attended twenty-five hours a week of classes in political science and foreign languages as preparation for going overseas in relief work. They were free to attend other classes at the university, and one subject completed his master's degree during the experiment. Many of them joined local churches and other organizations. They were also required to walk twenty-two miles a week, outdoors at their own pace, and another half hour on the treadmill. Each day, they walked two miles to get their meals from a university dining hall. During the control period and for the beginning months of semi-starvation, most chose to participate in activities such as ice-skating and folk dancing. In addition, they spent hours being examined physically and psychologically: testing math skills, memory retention, and hearing range; and giving interminable samples of blood, urine, stool, saliva, skin, sperm, and bone marrow.

For the first three months, the men ate an average of 3,500 calories a day, normal American fare, with 3.9 ounces of protein, 4.3 ounces of fat, and 17 ounces of carbohydrates. Each subject was to achieve his ideal weight by the end of the twelve weeks. Those who were too heavy got fewer calories; those who were too thin got more. As a group, the men ended this period slightly below their desired weight.

For the next six months, only two daily meals were served, at 8:30 a.m. and 5:00 p.m. Three menus were rotated, a monotonous diet of potatoes and whole wheat bread, cereal and cabbage, and turnips and rutabagas. On rare occasions, there were small portions of meat, sugar, milk, or butter. Daily calories averaged 1,570, with 1.7 ounces of protein and 1 ounce of fat. Individual body types had to be considered. Slighter, thinner men were expected to lose only 19 percent of their body weight and heavier men as much as 28 percent, with the goal being a group average of 24 percent. Daily and weekly adjustments in food were based on how well a man was achieving his predicted weight loss. If he were losing too much, he got extra potatoes and bread. If he were not losing enough, he got less.

Jim Graham was an idealistic twenty-two-year-old who had been planting trees and fighting forest fires before he joined the experiment. At that time, at 6'2", he weighed 175 pounds. "In the beginning," he remembered for an interview over thirty years later, "this was a rather interesting experience. We were losing weight, of course, but we still had a fair amount of energy."

Most of the men felt the same way, at least at first, although they complained of dizziness. Over the next few weeks, however, the experience became more painful.

The sensation of hunger increased; it never lessened. Eating habits began to change. The men became impatient waiting in line if the service was slow. They were possessive about their food. Some hunched over the trays, using their arms to protect their meal. Mostly they were silent, with the concentration that eating deserved. More and more men began to toy with their portions, mixing the items up, adding water, or "souping," to make new concoctions. They were liberal with the salt and asked for more spices. Dislikes for certain foods, such as rutabagas, disappeared. All food was eaten to the last bite. Then they licked their plates.

Obsessions developed around cookbooks and menus from local restaurants. Some men could spend hours comparing the prices of fruits and vegetables from one newspaper to the next. Some planned now to go into agriculture. They dreamed of new careers as restaurant owners.

One man had a harder time than the rest. Twenty-four years old, described as handsome, gregarious, and charming, he had seemed the perfect candidate. But in the first few weeks, he had disturbing dreams of "eating senile and insane people." As early as the third week, his weight showed discrepancies; he wasn't losing what he should be losing. One afternoon, in the eighth week of semi-starvation, his discipline broke down completely. Walking alone in town, he went into a shop and had an ice cream sundae, then another bowl of ice cream farther down the street, then a malted milk, then another. When he returned to the laboratory, he confessed. He felt awful. He had betrayed his own desire to "do service to a starving Europe and uphold the ideals of the Civilian Public Service program."

In response, the Minnesota researchers initiated the buddy system. No subject was allowed to go outside the laboratory, about town or around campus, without a friend or staff member. The men themselves understood the need. Those working in the kitchen asked to be reassigned.

The erring subject still felt badly. In truth, he really wanted to leave the experiment. But how could he admit that to himself and others? He violated his diet again, this time by stealing a few raw rutabagas. The writing in his daily journal was now an emotional swirl of ideas and prayers. He found some strength in God and decided to get a job in a grocery store to test himself. He couldn't sleep. He shoplifted some trinkets he didn't want. He rationalized his behavior to anyone who would listen, insisting that he was an individualist, that he wasn't meant for this kind of regimentation, that the experiment was a failure, that he had already done his share. He asked for a buddy to supervise him constantly. He gave up his money and checkbook. Finally he collapsed weeping,

threatening suicide and violence to others. The researchers released him from the experiment and admitted him to the psychiatric ward of the university hospital. What they termed a
borderline psychotic episode subsided after a few days.

Meanwhile another young man, twenty-five years old, was having
problems too. One night at a grocery store he ate two bananas, several cookies, and a sack of popcorn, all of which he vomited back up
at the laboratory. He referred to the incident as a "mental blackout."
For the next few weeks, he seemed confident and recommitted;
however, his weight failed to go down. Increasingly, he became rest-
less and unhappy but would not admit to any secret eating. At last,
he developed a urological problem and was released from the experiment. In retrospect, the researchers decided that the man had
"hysterical characteristics and other signs of a neurotic tempera-
ment. In interviews he was good-natured and easygoing but showed
signs of an immature Pollyanna attitude." They noted that every
other sentence in his journal ended with an exclamation point.

Eight weeks. Ten weeks. Twelve weeks. Sixteen weeks. Daily,
the physical changes in the Minnesota volunteers became more
dramatic. Prolonged hunger carves the body into what researchers call the asthenic build. The face grows thin, with pronounced cheekbones. Atrophied facial muscles may account for
the "mask of famine," a seemingly unemotional, apathetic stare.
The scrawny neck is pitiful. The clavicle looks sharp as a blade.
Broad shoulders shrink. Ribs are prominent. The scapular bones
in the back move like wings. The vertebral column is a line of
knobs. The knees are baggy, the legs like sticks. The fatty tissues
of the buttocks disappear, and the skin hangs in folds. The men
in the Minnesota laboratory now took a pillow with them everywhere they went because sitting had become uncomfortable.

The skeletal framework, however, seemed unchanged, something the researchers carefully measured. Populations in Russia and the Ukraine had reported a decrease in height during famine, but the Minnesota scientists found only an insignificant decline of .125 inches. They attributed the perceived larger decline to a weakening in muscle tone and posture. In five men, the researchers also measured the thickness of the spinal column's intervertebral disks and saw a loss of .04 inches. They speculated that changes in disk cartilage might be irreversible and could parallel the aging process.

"I felt like an old man," Jim Graham said, "and probably looked like one since I made no effort to stand up straight."

Edema complicated all kinds of measurements. Wrists and ankles might increase in circumference instead of decrease. Actual weight loss was obscured. The Minnesota scientists estimated that their subjects had as much as fourteen pounds of extra fluid after six months of semi-starvation. During refeeding, their height actually decreased as the swelling in their feet went down. Only four subjects showed no clinical signs of edema. Of the rest, many had fluid in their knee joints, which made walking painful. Jim Graham described how the men's flesh bulged over the tops of their shoes at the end of the day, and how his face was puffy in the morning, deeply marked with the indentations of his pillow. The men may have worsened their edema by using extra salt, drinking countless cups of tea or coffee, and watering their food in an effort to make a meal last longer. All this was accompanied by frequent urination during the day and night.

Their kidney functions remained normal.

Their resting metabolism was reduced by 40 percent, which the researchers estimated to be a savings of 600 calories a day.

Their hearts got smaller. After six months, with body weights reduced by 24 percent, the hearts of men like Jim Graham had shrunk by almost 17 percent. These hearts also beat slower, often very slow, and more regularly. Blood pressure dropped, except in five men, for whom it did not, and in one man, for whom it rose. Their veins sometimes collapsed now when blood was being drawn. The ability of the heart to work in general—the amount of blood pumped, the speed of blood, the arterial blood pressure—declined 50 percent. Electrocardiograms also showed less voltage and electrical energy, along with changes that pointed to possible heart damage. The researchers concluded that although this was abnormal, it was not serious. Semi-starvation did not include signs of heart disease or cardiac failure. (This would not have been true if the diet were deficient in thiamine or had fewer calories for a longer period of time, as with some anorectics.)

The ability of the lungs to bring in air decreased by 30 percent.

The brain and central nervous system seemed remarkably resistant. A battery of tests at the Minnesota laboratory showed little change in mental ability, although the men felt less intellectually active. They just didn't care as much. They lost their will for academic problems and became far more interested in cookbooks.

Two men developed neurological symptoms, such as numbness or burning and tingling. One wrote that his right foot felt unhinged at the ankle. The doctors decided that these feelings were hysterical in origin. They found it pertinent that a subject's numbness coincided with a new "numb" phase in his relationship with his ex-fiancée, who had broken up with him during the experiment. "No feeling aroused at all," the subject noted in his journal. "She might just as well have been any one of a dozen of other girls I know fairly well."

Generally, the men lost strength and endurance. In their jobs around the laboratory, they saw the difference. "Lifting the mattress off the bed to tuck the blankets in is a real chore," one man wrote, and "The carriers for the twelve urine bottles are a hell of a lot heavier than they used to be." Even personal hygiene became difficult. "I notice the weakness in my arms when I wash my hair in the shower; they become completely fatigued in the course of this simple operation." Or, "When the water in the showers becomes hot because of the flushing of the toilets, my reaction time in adjusting controls seems to be longer." It was wearying to walk upstairs, to carry things, to open a bottle of ink. Their handwriting got worse. Dressing took a long time. And they were clumsy, dropping books and tripping over their feet.

Their performance on the treadmill became an embarrassment to them. By the end of six months, the runs often ended in collapse. The researchers noted that the subjects did not stop because of shortness of breath or discomfort in the chest, as a heart patient might. They did not stop because of pain or nausea. "They stopped primarily because they could no longer control the actions of their knees and ankles. They literally did not have the strength to pick up their feet fast enough to keep up with the treadmill."

The men had no signs of vitamin deficiency, although the scientists emphasized how closely starvation can look like deficiency. During World War II, hungry populations in Europe did not generally suffer from beriberi, pellagra, scurvy, or rickets, perhaps due to their diet of vitamin-rich food, such as potatoes. But prisoners in Asia and the Pacific had a very different experience. They ate mostly polished rice, which lacks Vitamin A, and they commonly had a tropical disease, such as malaria, which may have had a synergistic effect. These men often had serious neurological damage and eye problems.

A third of the Minnesota volunteers complained that their hair, which seemed dry and stiff, "unruly and staring," was falling out. Their skin became scaly, a result of reduced blood flow. The area surrounding a hair follicle might turn hard and elevated, giving them a gooseflesh appearance and "nutmeg grater feel." Nineteen men had a brownish pigmentation around their mouth and under their eyes, deeper than any suntan. For two of the subjects, their long-term acne cleared up. Whenever they worked in the sun or had reason to sweat, all of the men developed tiny pockets of skin filled with perspiration, hundreds of plugged sweat ducts on their backs and shoulders.

Where not discolored, their skin was pale, with a distinctive grayish-blue pallor. As the blood circulating through their system became diluted with water, the proportion of red blood cells decreased by about 27 percent. The total amount of hemoglobin in their bodies decreased by 23 percent. In short, they were anemic.

They were also cold, even in that hot and humid July. Young men who had previously been fighting forest fires shivered in their beds under two or three woolen blankets. Their lips and nail beds turned blue. During the day, they wore jackets. Simultaneously, their tolerance for heat increased. They could hold hot plates easily and constantly begged for their food to be served at a higher temperature.

Their bone marrow lost healthy fat and had areas of "gelatinous degeneration."

Their eyesight remained normal. Their hearing improved. They had little tolerance for loud music and noisy conversation. They carried out their own discussions in quiet and subdued whispers.

Physically, the Minnesota volunteers now resembled the hungry populations of Europe. But there were important differences. The men living in the Laboratory of Physiological Hygiene did not suffer from the debilitating diarrhea so common in the Warsaw ghetto, in the concentration camps, and in most situations of famine and malnutrition. Nor did they experience much bloating, flatulence, or stomach pain. The researchers theorized that this was due to sanitation, the ready availability of soap and water, and "by the fact that the food served was not adulterated with bark, grass, leaves, sawdust, or even dirt, as is often the case when food is scarce." Unlike the people of Warsaw, the Minnesota subjects did not show an increase in cavities or loss in bone density, all of which may require a longer period of starvation. The Minnesota Experiment itself did not reproduce the cold that Europeans experienced in World War II, the lack of fuel for cooking food and heating the house, the lack of warm clothes, the lack of shoes. It did not reproduce the fear, the knowledge that you might die at any time, that you might be humiliated or injured or tortured or killed. It did not reproduce the murder of a neighbor, the corpses in the street, the inexplicable loss of human decency. It did not reproduce the death of your son.

"Above all," Jim Graham remembered, "we knew it would be over on a certain date."

And yet, despite the safety and normalcy of the lab, despite the knowledge that their ordeal would end in three months and then two months and then two weeks, the Minnesota volunteers felt it was their minds and souls that changed more than anything else. In many ways, they hardly recognized themselves. The lively, friendly group that had bonded together for the first months was now dull and apathetic, unwilling to plan activities or make decisions. They were rude to visitors and spent most of their time alone. It was "too much trouble" and too tiring to be with other people. The scientists mourned the loss of "the even-temperedness, patience, and tolerance" of the control period. Now the men indulged in outbursts of temper and emotion. They sulked and brooded and dramatized their discomforts. Those who deteriorated the most, socially and personally, were the most scorned. One man in particular became the group's scapegoat.

"We were no longer polite," Jim Graham said.

On excursions into town, always with a buddy, the men sometimes went on shopping sprees, possessed by the desire to collect knickknacks, second-hand clothes, and miscellaneous junk. Afterward, they were puzzled and dismayed: who would want these stacks of old books, this damaged coffee pot, this collection of spoons?

They were frequently depressed, although spells of elation could also come upon them suddenly, lasting a few hours to a few days. There was a "high" associated with the "quickening" effect of starvation and with the pride of successfully adapting to the diet. These high periods were followed by low ones, black moods, and feelings of discouragement.

Their behavior at the dinner table became more bizarre. While some men gulped down their meal like dogs at a food bowl, others lingered for hours, dawdling, noodling, stretching out the sensations.

Their sex drive diminished and then disappeared. "I have no more sexual feeling than a sick oyster," one declared. Some of the men had been dating, and that simply stopped. A few had other relationships in progress, and these became strained. One man was surprised at the new awkwardness, since he had thought his "friendship" was based solely on intellectual interests. When they went out to movies, the love scenes bored them, nothing was funny, and only scenes with food held their interest. Like the monks of earlier centuries, they no longer worried about nocturnal emissions or the desire to masturbate. Physically, their testes were producing fewer male hormones, and their sperm were less mobile and fewer in number.

On tests that measured mental health, the scores that concerned hypochondria, depression, and hysteria rose significantly. There were also increases in scores having to do with delusions and schizophrenia. The researchers regarded these changes as a "diffuse psychoneurosis." Their subjects had clearly become neurotic, a phenomenon that would reverse during refeeding. The symptoms of starvation neurosis were irritability, asociability, depression, nervousness, and emotional instability.

For the men who completed the experiment, there was no change in the area of psychosis—psychopathic behavior, paranoia, and hypomania (elevated moods or grandiosity). This was not true, however, for three of the four men who did not complete the experiment. Moreover, three out of thirty-six men chosen for their outstanding health and character would suffer some form of mental breakdown under the stress of hunger.

On May 26, 1945, about halfway through semi-starvation, a relief dinner was organized. One meal of twenty-three hundred calories was served. The men helped select the menu: roasted chicken and dressing, potatoes and gravy, strawberry shortcake. That night, the protein in the chicken triggered excessive water loss. Everyone got up even more than usual to urinate. The next day they discovered they had each lost several pounds.

Soon another subject was showing signs of distress. As early as the fifth week of semi-starvation, his weight loss had not followed the expected curve, and he confessed to minor violations, such as stealing and eating crusts of bread. He began to chew up to forty packs of gum a day, until his mouth was sore and he was caught stealing gum he could no longer afford. Throughout June and July, this twenty-five-year-old, described as a husky athlete, became increasingly nervous. He bought an old suit he didn't need and later wailed, "Nobody in his right mind would do a thing like that." He talked often of his compulsion to root through garbage cans. Later interviews would reveal he was doing just that, although at the time he didn't confess to breaking the diet. Despite cuts in his daily calories, his weight failed to reach a loss of 24 percent, and he was released from the experiment. His neurotic behavior continued with cycles of overeating and illness. At one point, he committed himself to the psychiatric ward of the university hospital but did not stay for treatment. In a meeting with the psychologists, he wept and kicked over a table. He couldn't make simple decisions and was painfully disgusted with himself. The researchers believed optimistically that his problems would eventually subside.

This man had a close friend who followed a similar pattern, becoming addicted to gum chewing, and failing to lose the prescribed weight. He also denied eating extra food and appeared extremely depressed. His data was not used in the research, although he remained at the laboratory. Another subject in these last few weeks of semi-starvation expressed the fear that he was going crazy. Yet another admitted how close he came to hitting a man over the head with his dinner tray.

By now, the education program at the laboratory had ended for lack of interest. There were no more seminars in foreign languages or relief work. Housekeeping chores were neglected. The working schedule of fifteen hours a week had long since slipped into half-hearted efforts. Some regular exercise was still maintained; at least, the men continued to walk back and forth to the dining hall.

Six months had come to seem like an eternity, with each day stretching infinitely long. Finally, at long last, the longed-for day arrived, July 29, 1945, the end of semi-starvation and the beginning of the twelve-week rehabilitation period. It was Jim Graham's twenty-third birthday. The men felt like cheering. "Morale was high," Jim Graham said. The worst was over.

In fact, it was not. The goal of the Minnesota Experiment had been to determine how to refeed a starving population with the most economical use of food, assuming that a minimum of resources would be available. In other words, what was the least you could give a starving man and still have him recover? The remaining thirty-two men were now randomly divided into four groups. One group, for the first six weeks, received four hundred more calories a day, the next group eight hundred more calories, the third group twelve hundred more calories, and the last group sixteen hundred more calories. Those in the first group got about two thousand daily calories and those in the highest about three thousand. These four groups were each further subdivided into two, with half receiving extra protein in the form of soybean powder added into their bread. The protein subgroups were divided again, with half each receiving a vitamin supplement and the other half a placebo.

In all cases, the rehabilitation diet meant the same kind of food, just more of it. Surprisingly, that wasn't a bad thing. "They warned us that the food would get monotonous," Jim remembered. "But it was far from monotonous. It was food and any food tasted good. To this day, I find the tastiest food a simple boiled potato."

In the first weeks of refeeding, a number of men started losing water and weight. Edema had masked their degree of starvation; now it masked their degree of recovery. These men found the weight loss disturbing. Moreover, a very slow weight gain was seen in all the groups, especially in the men given fewer calories. By the sixth week, the first group had gained an insignificant 0.3 percent of the weight lost during semi-starvation. Essentially they looked much the same: skeletal, hollow-cheeked, morose. The second group gained back 9.1 percent of the weight lost, the third group 11.1 percent, and the fourth group, getting as much as three thousand calories a day, only 19.2 percent. Their blood sugar level increased only slightly. Their blood pressure and pulse rate remained low. They still felt tired and depressed. They still had the sex drive of a sick oyster. They still had edema. They still had aches and pains. And they still felt hungry. Some felt even hungrier than before.

One twenty-eight-year-old had begun the experiment as a leader, but in the last six months, this "highly intelligent" and "engaging" personality had become one of the weakest and most aggravating members of the group. He spent hours making disgusting messes of his food, and his air of suffering irritated everyone. On the last day, July 28, he collapsed on the treadmill, which caused him to sob uncontrollably. For this subject, assigned to the group receiving the next to lowest calories, the letdown of refeeding was unbearable. At the end of the first week, while changing a tire, he allowed his automobile to slip the jack. One finger was almost torn off and required outpatient care at the university hospital. The man confessed he had deliberately attempted to mutilate himself but had lost his nerve at the last moment and had done an incomplete job.

The next week, the young man visited a friend and went into the yard to chop wood for the fire, something he had done before. This time he also chopped off three of his fingers. During a five-day stay in the hospital, he explained, "When rehabilitation started, I was still hungry. It was really more starvation. . . . I was blue over the whole thing. I was in a weird frame of mind." Seemingly, his only option was to get out of the Civilian Public Service altogether. So, "I decided to get rid of some fingers."

The Minnesota researchers convinced the subject to stay in the experiment, and during his time in the hospital, his calories remained at the prescribed level, although he received new kinds of food, such as fruit. He returned to the lab refreshed, ready to complete the refeeding stage. The scientists theorized that the extra care had substituted for the "mothering" his immature personality required. The subject now repressed the memory that his mutilation had been deliberate, arguing that his muscle strength and control had been weak or that the ax had hit a branch. He also developed an aversion to the psychology tests and to the psychologists in the experiment. This puzzled him.

By the end of the sixth week of refeeding, almost all the subjects were in active rebellion. Many "grew argumentative and negativistic." Some questioned the value of the project, as well as the motives and competence of the researchers. A few admitted that their desire to help the relief effort had completely disappeared. At the same time, unnoticed by the subjects themselves, their energy was returning. They became more responsive, albeit in a negativistic way. They were annoyed at the restrictions still imposed on them. They rejected the buddy system, which was removed "in the face of imminent wholesale violation." They resisted going back to a regular work schedule. At times, the experimenters felt they were watching "an overheated boiler, the capacity of the safety values an unknown variable."

Later, the researchers compared this with what they learned about refeeding camps after the war, where aid workers also noted a growing aggressiveness and surprising "lack of gratitude" in men and women who had previously been dull and apathetic with hunger.

Now all four groups got an increase of another eight hundred calories and the supplemented group another .84 ounces of protein. Slowly, more slowly than expected, their hearts increased in size. The capacity of the lungs improved. The brown pigmentation of the skin began to fade, and the acne that had disappeared came back.

In another four weeks, everyone got an additional 259 calories and the protein group another boost. At the end of the experiment, the group with the least calories was eating an average of three thousand a day and the group with the most as much as four thousand. Their weight gains were still only 21 percent of weight lost for the lowest group and 57 percent for the highest group. Most of the weight gain was in body fat, not muscle mass. The more calories a man got, the more fat and the greater percentage of fat he gained.

The souping of meals, the excessive drinking of fluids and use of salt, and the obsessive interest in food continued. Table manners were shocking.

After three months of refeeding, the groups taking extra vitamins did not seem to have benefited in any way. Nor had the groups taking extra protein. The supplements did not help increase red blood cell count or metabolism. They did not help in the recovery of normal blood pressure and pulse rate or in the return of strength and endurance and general fitness. In fact, the men who did not receive protein supplements recovered their grip strength faster than those who did.

The men receiving extra calories did benefit. They gained weight faster. Their blood pressure, resting metabolism, strength, and endurance rose more quickly. Their fitness scores improved, and they were better able to do work. The rate of recovery for starvation neurosis, particularly depression and hysteria, was directly linked to how much food was in the new diet. More calories made a man feel better physically and psychologically.

By now, the war was over. Germany had surrendered in May 1945 and Japan in August. Dr. Ancel Keys, director of the Laboratory and of the Minnesota Experiment, offered some preliminary advice in terms of what the scientists had learned about refeeding. First, the allies needed to physically rehabilitate the starved people of Europe before talking to them about democracy. Giving these people extra vitamins or protein would not necessarily be helpful. And no real rehabilitation could take place on two thousand calories a day; the proper diet was more like four thousand.

By the end of the experiment, almost one year after it had begun, the Minnesota volunteers were far from normal, but they were on their way. Their humor and social skills had somewhat returned, and they were looking forward to the future. Twelve subjects agreed to stay on at the laboratory for another eight weeks of testing. Now they were allowed to eat whatever they wanted. A few celebrated by consuming as much as ten thousand calories a day. Many had the sensation of being hungry even after they had just eaten a large meal; some would eat three lunches in a row. Others felt anxious that food would be taken away. Jim Graham carried candy bars and cookies in his pockets, so he would have something to eat whenever he wanted.

The influx of food seemed to overload the system. Most men had some new form of discomfort, from bloating and heartburn to shortness of breath and sleepiness. Five men still had swollen knees and feet, sometimes worse than before. Now the atrophic, weakened heart showed its vulnerability, not in semi-starvation but in rehabilitation. One subject, eating between seven thousand and ten thousand calories a day for a week, had signs of cardiac failure—difficulty breathing, a puffy face, pitting edema, and an enlarged heart. After bed rest, a reduced diet, and reduced salt, the symptoms disappeared.

Eventually, four months after the end of starvation, almost everyone had returned to a more moderate daily intake of thirty-two hundred to forty-two hundred calories. By now they had all surpassed their pre-starvation weight, and the researchers commented that a "soft roundness became the dominant characteristic" of men who had entered the experiment lean and fit. By the end of five months, their sex drive had returned and their sperm were vigorous and motile. Their hearts were normal sized. Their lung capacities were normal. Over eight months later, the researchers were still monitoring sixteen of the subjects. Most had no complaints except for shortness of breath. Most were overweight. Jim Graham had ballooned from his control weight of 175 to 225, and he would continue to gain. One man still felt physically lethargic. One still had some edema. Those who had complained of nervousness felt better. Their eating habits were close to acceptable.

. . .

The changes in the Minnesota volunteers highlighted the effect of nutrition on the human body. This so impressed the director of the experiment, Dr. Ancel Keys, that he went on to direct two long-term studies that looked at diet, one on Minnesota businessmen and one that followed the health of men in sixteen populations in seven countries. Ancel Keys knew that the rate of heart attacks had fallen in Europe during World War II when meat and dairy products were less available. His research implicated bloodstream cholesterol in heart disease. He confirmed that saturated fat helped determine cholesterol levels and populations that ate less saturated fat had fewer heart attacks. Keys went on to write a popular book promoting "The Mediterranean Diet" and was instrumental in convincing nutritionists that they could make big changes in public health. Americans began to look at their butter and steak differently. The debate about food would never be the same.

THE ANTHROPOLOGY
OF HUNGER

WE KNOW A MODEST AMOUNT ABOUT HOW hunger shapes the human body, especially in a select group of young men in a highly controlled environment. Hunger also shapes human culture, and we have tried to understand this as well. To some extent, the anthropology of hunger has been a taboo subject or, at least, a problematic one. We are reluctant to admit hunger as a norm. We are surprised and repelled at what people do when they are hungry. And we are profoundly irresolute about our own response: what is our responsibility to large groups of hungry people?

In the 1930s, Audrey Richards studied nutrition in the Bantu and Bemba tribes of Rhodesia. She showed how behavior such as listlessness accompanied the "hungry season" just before the rains. She noted a change in food-sharing. People were less generous, even to family members.

In 1941, Allan Holmberg went to live with the nomadic, hunting and gathering Siriono Indians of eastern Bolivia, a functional culture that had long suffered from food shortage. Holmberg found in them a "hunger frustration" that had evolved into a hasty preparation of food and a lack of complex recipes. There were few routines, rituals, or courtesies around a meal. Instead, people stole off into the forest to eat or wolfed what they had. They were reluctant to share and had few food preferences "except on a quantitative basis." They overate, they ate when they were not hungry, and they ate when they were sick. There was also "excessive quarrelling over food, fantasies and dreams about food, and insults in terms of food."

In this society, children were freely given their mother's breast and did not experience hunger until weaned. After that, parents showed a child "greater love" when it was suffering from hunger. Although the Sirionos abandoned aged and sick adults, they nurtured and protected even deformed children (15 percent of the tribe had a club foot, due to inbreeding). Marriage practices, prestige, and magical rituals almost always had something to do with food. Sex was easily obtained with a promise of food, although in times of extreme scarcity, people showed little interest in sex. Otherwise, intercourse was frequent not only for married couples but also between a husband and his wife's sisters, and a wife and her husband's brothers, and between other tribal members "classified" as sisters or brothers or potential husbands or potential wives. Premarital sex was encouraged, the best partner being young and plump. Holmberg concluded, "While food often compensates for sex deprivation in our own society, among the Siriono love appears frequently to serve as a compensation for hunger."

In a very different situation, the sedentary Gurage people of southwest Ethiopia also showed signs of hunger frustration. When William and Dorothy Shack studied this group in the early 1960s, the Gurage had depended for generations on the abundant, year-

round *ensete,* or "false banana plant," supplemented by grains, vegetables, cheese, butter, and meat. Famine and starvation were
then unknown, but damage to crops through warfare had been a
historical reality. Still, the Gurage had sophisticated methods of
crop rotation, transplanting, storage, and food production. The
Shacks believed that most Gurage grew and stored far more food
than their families could use. Commonly, they hid excess supplies
of *ensete* in underground pits, sometimes for years, where the vegetable rotted and went to waste. The hunger anxiety of the Gurage
did not seem to come from their environment, the Shacks wrote,
so much as from "values placed on hoarding and self-denial which
prevent the daily satiation of hunger."

Meals in a Gurage household were susceptible to uninvited,
unexpected guests who had to be fed under the rules of hospitality. These meals were usually small and inadequate. People com-
pensated by eating most of their food late at night, secretly,
privately, in a darkened hut, surrounded only by close family
members. Slenderness in males and females was prized and
overeating considered vulgar. One exception involved a show of
gluttony at monthly ceremonies or religious rituals. Also, an illness in which a Gurage seemed possessed by an evil spirit was
cured by having the patient cover himself with a blanket and stuff
his mouth with specially prepared food.

The Shacks theorized that the Gurage anxiety around food
began in infancy. Until being weaned at the age of two to four,
Gurage children mainly received breast milk. But the experience
of breastfeeding was unsatisfying, with mothers often absent or
busy or unresponsive. If the breast were available, the child usually engaged in "a constant struggle to keep the mother's nipple in
its mouth" while she continued, in a harried way, to churn milk or

card raw cotton. During the day, babies were laid down and left to cry from hunger or lack of attention. Older children were fed haphazardly, after the adults. The Gurage treated males differently than females, with brothers fed first and supposedly more, their sisters being required to prepare and serve food for them. Yet boys seemed to develop a greater hunger anxiety, perhaps because girls had more access to food since they controlled its preparation.

The Shacks observed qualities they thought related to the Gurage culture of hunger. The Gurage were "selfish" and carefully calculated the reciprocity expected of any gift. They stayed emotionally detached from family members and expressed a relationship mainly in terms of obligations. They were passive. When confronted with a problem, a Gurage often said, "What can we do? We can do nothing." They had feelings of worthlessness and needed constant reassurances that their land or food or culture was as good as those of other Ethiopians.

In the 1970s, another anthropologist, Michael Young, described the food anxiety of the Kalauna people in Papua New Guinea. Similar to the Gurage, these Melanesians had plenty of food most of the time, although they had lived historically with drought and famine. Like the Gurages, they admired thinness and "a small tight stomach" and abhorred gluttony. They also practiced denial. In the planting season, men and women ate nothing during the day but worked on an empty stomach, chewing betel nuts or smoking tobacco to mitigate their hunger. Almost always they ate privately. Unlike the Gurage, they did not balance their frugal meals with ceremonies of overeating.

The Kalaunans had important magic rituals intended to help the people by making them anorexic—denying their need for and pleasure in food. As a sorcerer walked through the vegetable gardens, chanting spells, spitting betel juice, and inspecting the crops, he did so with "undesiring eyes," indifferent to the bounty of the harvest. Later, the women who weeded the gardens would follow the sorcerer's example, their eyes also "nondesiring, their bellies tight and contented, their hands restrained, so that, like model housewives, they will not be tempted to gather more than the minimum needed for the family meal." Similar to the Gurage, the Kalaunans preferred to have food rot in the garden or in storage rather than be consumed gluttonously.

Other magic involved "fighting with hunger." A particularly feared curse made the victim feel hungry even though he or she had just eaten. That person might then steal food from another person's garden. In her shameful hunger, her grabbing and gobbling, she might eat so much that her stomach would burst and she would die. The worst magic a sorcerer could do was to inflict this craving on an entire community. When Michael Young visited the Kalaunans in 1979, he found them currently under that threat: the community had just been cursed and their stomachs were feeling ominously empty.

For eighteen months in 1965–66, anthropologist Colin Turnbull conducted the most famous and controversial study of how hunger shapes culture, this time on some two thousand Africans called Ik, who were living and starving near the northern border of Uganda and Kenya. The Ik were prevented from hunting in the nearby national park and forcibly confined to patches of infertile land. Turnbull estimated that their natural patterns of hunting, foraging, and farming had been disrupted since the 1930s and probably before that. He believed that the Ik's adaptation to long-term hunger was to abandon social relationships and institutions, even familial ones. Literally, it was every man—and every woman and child—for himself. Husbands did not share with wives, nor wives with husbands, nor parents with children, nor children with parents. Cooperation became maladaptive. Only the strong, the selfish, and the predatory survived.

Turnbull described a family unit hardly recognizable to the rest of the world. With reluctance and anger, a mother nursed her child for the first two years. In the third year, the toddler was weaned, a deliberate breaking of emotional and physical bonds that, Turnbull wrote, "seemed excessive and brutal at times." In fact, the cruelty of adults was an important part of the child's education: "In this way a responsible Ik mother taught her child, as best she could, the value of independence." At three years of age, children were thrown out of the house, allowed only to sleep in the outside compound. On their own, without food or shelter, they joined a gang of other children whose ages went up to seven or eight. If they survived the next few years through foraging or stealing from the fields and gardens, they joined a second gang of older children—big enough now to climb the wild fig trees. At twelve or thirteen, they were fully mature and continued the search for food alone. Turnbull stressed that the child-gangs served mainly to protect the children from thieving adults, and children were the most ruthless and vicious of the Ik, tormenting the weak among them, as well as the elderly in the village.

The elderly, like any weakened Ik, went unfed until they died. Usually they crept into abandoned huts where they starved to death alone. Turnbull began to feed a few of these elders and caused excitement whenever he appeared; hopeful, the old people would drag themselves to the doorways to attract his attention. "To enter into any village," he wrote in 1966, "is like entering a graveyard, skeletons crawling about trying to pick up a grain that has

fallen from the baskets of their healthy offspring." Often the anthropologist found himself protecting an old man from a group of
teasing children or running off an adult stealing food he had just
given a dying woman. The Ik strongly disapproved of "this waste."
Old people "had no eyes or legs." They were already dead. (An elderly Ik could be anyone over the age of thirty. Similarly, the literature from World War II is full of scenes in which malnourished
adults are mistaken for men and women twice their age.)

The people Turnbull cared about were precisely the ones who did
not fit into such a society. Adupa was a bony, emaciated thirteen-
year-old girl with a distended stomach. Her unusual qualities of
innocence and kindness only made her vulnerable. When the
other children stole her food and hit her, "Adupa cried," Turnbull
believed, "not because of the pain in her body, but because of the
pain she felt at that great vast empty wasteland where love should
have been." Moved, the anthropologist began feeding Adupa as
well, "probably the cruelest thing I have ever done" since it only
prolonged the child's misery. Above all, Adupa wanted to be with
her parents and kept returning to their compound. Exasperated,
they finally brought her into the house and then left, closing the
hut tightly so the weakened girl could not escape. When they returned a week later, their daughter was dead, and they threw her
into a nearby ravine, covering the body with a layer of stones.

There was no burial rite for Adupa or for most of the deaths
Turnbull observed. The Ik seemed to have few remaining ceremonies or rituals. In Turnbull's account, marriage was a bleak,
loveless affair—mainly a way to get help in building a house. Adul-
tery and wife-beating were common. People preferred solitary
lives. They hunted alone, gathered food alone, and always tried to
eat alone. Sometimes, Turnbull did see Ik men come together and

sit for hours, staring at a view of their sacred mountain, saying nothing, doing nothing. He also saw the need for human contact when the hunger was at its worst, as people gathered in silent clusters, crawling to join other Ik in a group. Turnbull described their progress as they squatted first, raised their buttocks, and then propelled themselves forward on their arms, skin folds flapping. He marveled, "They just wanted to be with others, and they stopped whenever they met."

The Ik often took pleasure in the misfortunes of others. They could be equally humorous about their own problems. In one story, Turnbull shook hands with an old man, weighing about sixty pounds, who then tightened his grip and was pulled off the ground as Turnbull moved away. The old man collapsed, laughing, and held out his hand again, still laughing, for Turnbull to help him back to a sitting position. The Ik apologized for his behavior, saying that he hadn't eaten for three days and so it was difficult for him to stand up, "Whereupon he and his companion dissolved into laughter again."

Years later, in a paper called "Rethinking the Ik," Turnbull concluded, "Since the Ik have revised their concept of normality to fit their present context they do not see themselves as being under stress. Even young people dying of starvation seem remarkably well adjusted to their situation and see nothing abnormal about it."

In his book *The Mountain People*, the anthropologist's relationship with the Ik seemed hostile from the beginning. His earlier work had been with the Congo pygmies who had welcomed him into their forest society and who he idealized in return. He had not wanted to study the little-known, mountain-loving Ik but had no other field opportunities. His first impressions of his Ik guides were negative. These people didn't seem to like him either. They lied to him, stole from him, and manipulated him whenever possible. Ironically, Turnbull had little understanding of how hunger affects people. He often wondered why the Ik were not more interested in sex, and he was slow to notice the extent of the starvation around him.

Soon, he began to mirror what he described as Ik behavior. He retreated to his Land Rover to cook and eat his meals alone, while hungry Ik huddled and waited outside. He hoarded his medical supplies, flying into a rage when a visiting friend gave an anti-dysentery tablet to a sick child. (Recounting this story to a journalist, and recalling that he had a thousand more tablets for his own use, Turnbull confessed, "At that moment, I stopped and suddenly realized I didn't care about these people at all. If they died, it was just fodder for my notebook.") Like the Ik, he also began to enjoy and make fun of other people's misfortunes. When a particularly nasty boy was beaten by his sisters, Turnbull described a sense of pleasure as he listened to the child's shrieks. His relationship with his informant Atum became increasingly hateful. On one trip, "The unpleasantness of returning was somewhat alleviated by Atum's suffering on the way up the stony trail. Several times he slipped, which made Lojieri and me laugh."

In a *New Yorker* interview, Turnbull admitted that he could not empathize with the Ik the way an anthropologist should. "They are starving to death all around me. I see them getting weaker and weaker. Since they're not allowed to leave Uganda, they can't follow the game. As long as I have enough to eat, I can't identify with them. I live on rice and lentils, and I give them what I can, but I can't support two thousand people."

At the close of *The Mountain People*, Turnbull wrote, "I knew that the Ik as a society were almost certainly finished, and that the monster they had created in its place, that passionless, feelingless association of individuals, would continue, spreading like a fungus, contaminating all it touched. When I left, I too had been contaminated." Nothing proved this point more than when Ugandan authorities asked Turnbull for advice on what to do with the Ik. He suggested rounding them up, separating family members, and dispersing random groups of less than ten to different mountain regions. In this way, the hunger-created culture of the Ik would be completely destroyed.

The Mountain People became a best seller, a widely read book still in print today. Turnbull appeared on national talk shows, and the head of the Royal Shakespeare Company adapted the story of the Ik into a popular play. That story, of course, was really about us: what human beings could and would do under the stress of hunger.

If lay readers seemed fascinated and moved by *The Mountain People*, many anthropologists were appalled. They criticized Turnbull for being excessively judgmental, unprofessional, and gullible. A new concern—one that no one had faced before—was how to study subjects who are starving and in need of immediate help. In an article called "On Responsibility and Humanity: Calling a Colleague to Account," Fredrik Barth pointed to Turnbull's "egocentric response" in feeding his favorite Ik on daily food rounds that included some and excluded others. Turnbull's selfishness and hostility were seen as a kind of Stockholm syndrome in which he became what he studied. Another report on the Ik in 1980 pointed to more problems in Turnbull's work. His former informants now said that the anthropologist's understanding of their language had been poor, that he had gotten most of his information from non-Ik, and that much of that information was false. Appalled at Turnbull's description of them, the Ik threatened that if he ever returned to their mountain region, they would "force him to eat his own feces." Although this report defended the Ik as a functional culture, it did not refute Turnbull's descriptions of child-rearing or the abandonment of the weak in time of hunger.

In a private letter, Colin Turnbull responded to Barth's comments with the suggestion that his colleague had been "somewhat unhinged by the Ik." In truth, it seemed that Colin Turnbull had been unhinged, unprepared for the complexity of a long-term, slow-motion famine in which some people starved and others did not, in which outside aid was inefficient and abused, in which all kinds of people behaved very badly—and all these deaths just didn't make sense, not when you came from a culture of abundance, not when restaurants and cinemas and hospitals were a plane ride away. You looked around, noting that only the selfish and predatory survived, and then you realized you were a survivor. You were not one of the good guys. The good guys were dead.

To his credit, Turnbull did try to secure famine relief for the Ik and he did try to save individuals. For his Western readers, he painted the darkest face of hunger, and he drew us into that picture. "Most of us are unlikely to admit readily that we can sink as low as the Ik," he wrote, "but many of us do, and with far less cause."

. . .

Anthropologist Robert Dirk looked at large-scale social responses to food shortage and described three common phases. Once the threat is noticed, there is general alarm. People are excited and may become more gregarious. They may share more, setting up such things as communal kitchens. They may migrate. Emotions increase. There is irritability and anger, political unrest, possible rioting, and looting. There may be more religious ritual, increased devotion, and mystical acts.

In the second stage, resistance is directed against the hunger itself, as opposed to its cause. People conserve energy rather than expend it. They are less social, their actions focused on obtaining food. Small, closed groups, such as the family unit, become the most effective way to survive. Friends and extended family may need to be excluded. Stealing is common. Organized political work diminishes, although there may be random acts of aggression and violence. In this social disorder, people turn more trustingly to authority. Dirk noted that this happened twelve weeks into the Minnesota Experiment when the subjects asked for more restrictions and controls for their behavior.

The last phase is marked by a collapse of all cooperative efforts, even within the family. This can happen gradually. The elderly are the first to be sacrificed and then young children. People become physically as well as emotionally exhausted, sitting for long hours, staring at nothing, saying nothing. Much of what Turnbull described among the Ik is a portrait of a people in this third stage.

Individuals, however, do not always follow the larger pattern. Disaster, Dirk wrote, "brings out the very best and the very worst in people; it exaggerates what is already there." Among the Ik, Turnbull saw a few children like Adupa, and a few adults who managed to survive despite their maladaptive kindness. In any extreme situation, there will be heroic gestures that have nothing to do with maximizing survival. There will be men and women who choose to die rather than betray their child, their parent, their friend, their community, or their personal belief.

The specific culture and history of a society can also affect how that society responds to famine. Even in a severe food shortage, the

Ik apparently did not practice cannibalism. But in Ukrainian villages in the famine of 1932–33, in which five to eight million Ukrainians died when farms were collectivized and grain seized by the government, people and corpses mysteriously disappeared. The authorities put up stern posters, "Eating dead children is barbarism," and transferred all cases of cannibalism to the secret police. Similarly, in the 1941 Siege of Leningrad, when the city struggled to live on declining food rations, frozen bodies in the street often showed flesh sliced from the buttocks or legs. About two thousand people were arrested during the siege for eating other people. Some Russians believed that cannibalism had become organized, with criminal groups systematically kidnapping and butchering their victims.

The biggest famine in recorded history also took place in the middle of the twentieth century, also involved cannibalism, and also was entirely man made. In 1958, when Chairman Mao Ze-Dong wanted China to become a great industrial nation, he ordered millions of peasants to neglect their fields and smelt unusable steel by melting down their cooking pots and tools. When he wanted China to become a great producer of grain, he collectivized the peasants' farms and insisted on unscientific methods of growing crops that inadvertently reduced production. Under intense pressure, peasants and officials competed to grow the most food. Harvests were reported at twice, three times, a hundred times their actual yield. Delighted with these inflated numbers, Mao and the party took a percentage of the grain to be stored near urban centers. Sometimes that percentage was the entire real harvest, leaving nothing for the people in the countryside. At the same time, China cut its imports of food and doubled its exports. As people began to starve, Mao ignored them. Any sign of famine was blamed on treacherous "criminals" who were hoarding grain.

Hundreds of thousands of people were put into prison where they died as surely as if they had been allowed to stay home.

China had always been a land of hunger. Records document 1,828 famines from 108 BC to AD 1911 Governing officials developed ways to handle these emergencies, from ritual ceremonies and sacrifices to storing surplus food in state-owned granaries. The peasants also adopted strategies and passed down methods of survival, a famine culture of when to migrate away from your home, when to sell your children as slaves or prostitutes, how to make flour from dirt and leaves, and which plants are edible and which poisonous. Cannibalism was another social response, as it was in the major famines of Europe and elsewhere. Chinese historian Key Ray Chong pointed to the sixth century BC when an observer of a siege wrote, "In the city, we are exchanging our children and eating them and splitting up their bodies for fuel." Three hundred years later, when perhaps half the population of China was dying of hunger, the emperor officially decreed that parents could also sell or eat their children.

In his book *Hungry Ghosts*, journalist Jasper Becker wrote that after the fall of 1959, with grain production in China dropping lower and lower, cannibalism became widespread. The state still insisted on taking its quota and began seizing not just grain but livestock and vegetables. In the destitute villages, all that people had left was the thin gruel served by communal kitchens. "Generally," Becker wrote, "the villagers ate the flesh of corpses, especially those of children. In rare cases, parents ate their own children, elder brothers ate younger brothers, elder sisters ate younger sisters." In the area of Anhui, people still used the proverb, *Yi zi er shi*, or "Swap child, make food." One of Becker's interviewers described how "They stopped giving the girl children food. They just gave them water. They swapped the body of their daughter with that of a neighbor's. . . . Then they boiled the corpses into a kind of soup. People had learned to do this during the famine of the 1930s. People accepted this as a kind of hunger culture." Becker found similar stories about cannibalism from all parts of China, documented in police reports, in prison writings, and in party records.

Many Chinese described the physical signs of hunger—waterlogged skin like doughy bread, constant urination, diarrhea, bleeding and brittle nails, and deep cracks in the hands and feet. Writer Zhang Xianliang, a prisoner in a labor camp, remembered the death masks of men who were about to die, how the skin of their faces and bodies turned a "dull, dark color; their hair looked dried-out and scorched; the mucus of their eyes increased but the eyes themselves became exceedingly, strangely bright. They emitted a 'thief's glare,' a kind of shifty, scared yet crafty, debilitated but also poisonous light." Sometimes the prisoners experienced a sudden burst of energy and spirit, their cheeks turning rosy, "the last redness of the setting sun." He described the edema that made a man resemble "a balloon that had been filled full of air—the eyes would swell until they became small slits; light couldn't penetrate them and one could not see out."

By the end of 1960, even the cities suffered from a lack of food since few farmers had had the strength to plant new crops. Migration was prohibited, and people were dying in villages only a few miles outside Beijing. Meanwhile, in many areas, the grain stored by the state was left to rot. Some people rebelled, with desperate attacks on granaries and trains. But the peasants—weakened with hunger, unarmed, and poorly organized—had little chance against the militia. Apathy became the prevalent response, following Dirk's pattern of alarm, resistance, and exhaustion.

Entire villages or half of village populations perished. The prisons were death camps, although in some cases prisoners escaped only to find even less food in the surrounding areas. Finally, as more soldiers and party members received news of their families dying at home, a few leaders defied Mao and began reforms, which revived agricultural production. By fall 1962, people in the cities were getting a minimum of food. Still, Becker reported that in some places women did not menstruate again until 1965 and among peasants "hunger remained endemic" for decades.

In a few years, Mao's Cultural Revolution would purge those party members who had set up the reforms that ended the starvation. Outside China, no one guessed at the extent of the disaster until the mid-1980s when China released census data that researchers could match with other accounts. Thirty to forty million people had starved to death. In 1980, the notes of dissident Wei Jingsheng were smuggled out of China and published in the *New York Times*, "During a gathering at a friend's house in the neighboring village, I heard horror stories of villagers who had exchanged babies to eat. I pitied them all. Who had made these parents live to taste, inconceivably, of human flesh mixed with parental tears?"

. . .

In 1992, anthropologist Nancy Scheper-Hughes published *Death Without Weeping: The Violence of Everyday Life in Brazil*, an effort to integrate biology (the research of the Minnesota Experiment) into a long-term study of hunger in Brazilian cane workers, whose calorie level has been estimated to fall as low as fifteen hundred to seventeen hundred a day. Scheper-Hughes praised Colin Turnbull for breaking "the taboo of silence on hunger" and for highlighting "the fragility of all social life and social institutions, even that most sacred of all sacred cows, the family." Although the chronically undernourished cane workers in northern Brazil had some parallels to the Ik, the observations of their anthropologist would be infinitely more compassionate.

Scheper-Hughes believed that after the 1970s, hunger and food shortage began to interest anthropologists more. They confined their interpretations to two main camps. The bio-ecological model emphasized how people physically responded to malnutrition and how these effects—stunting, infertility, and infant mortality—could be seen as an adaptation to declining resources or population pressure. The second camp focused on the symbolic and metaphoric meaning of food, food taboos, and hunger. In both cases, hungry people remained subjects of study, and the personal reality of hunger was kept at a comfortable, academic distance.

Nancy Scheper-Hughes began her study of hunger as a twenty-year-old Peace Corps worker in a community of five thousand rural workers called Alto do Cruzeiro. In 1964, she was sent to a local health care clinic—which few people visited or trusted—and then moved on to become a *visitadora*, actively taking her bag of immunizations and medical supplies into people's homes, where she was welcomed. During the drought of 1965, she saw "a veritable die out of Alto babies," children clearly malnourished, starving, and dehydrated. The mystery was not why the children were dying, for that seemed obvious, but why the mothers were so indifferent to these deaths and so willing to see them as natural, a product of the child's unwillingness to eat, his aversion to life, or his weak spirit.

At first, the health worker was devastated. She wept as she carried the tiny body to its mother. Gradually she realized that her sorrow was not being shared. Over the twenty-five years she visited the Brazilian community, she learned that these deaths were so common as to be expected. These babies were only "visitors," frail "little birds," potential angels soon buried in a cardboard coffin at a funeral that rarely involved grief—a death without weeping. Mother love and maternal bonding had been suspended in this hungry culture until the child proved its strength and willingness for life. This suspension could be self-fulfilling as listless, anemic children were neglected and ignored. Such children were condemned from the beginning by signs of paleness or passivity or emaciation. Scheper-Hughes learned that part of being a mother in Alto do Cruzeiro included knowing when to let go of a child who "showed" that he wanted to die. "The other part is knowing just when it is safe to let oneself go enough to love a child, to trust him or her to be willing to enter the *luta* (struggle) that is this life on earth."

Overwhelmed by poverty, hunger, and disease, the people of the Alto saw themselves as weak and helpless. Because Alto mothers felt their own breast milk was also weak and worthless (especially the watery, bluish colostrum that first nourishes a newborn) the culture of breastfeeding was replaced by bottle-feeding and a complicated array of formulas, either too expensive to buy in enough quantity or too poor in quality to nourish a child. Moreover, the artificial milk was usually mixed with unclean water. As a result, young babies often sickened and starved. Older siblings who had managed to survive usually went hungry too, in households that commonly didn't have enough food, where adults and children alike drank sugar water and went to sleep hoping tomorrow would be better.

In Brazil, an industrialized country that exported food, with the world's eighth largest economy, Scheper-Hughes described the madness of the last stages of hunger, *delirio de fome*, something long known in Brazilian literature and folk tradition. She cared for one little boy, "an hour-long delirium in which the child went rigid, seemed to buckle, and then finally became wild, growling and snapping at our ministering hands until, thankfully, he died." The Alto people referred to such deaths as the dog's disease, likening hunger madness to the madness of rabies.

Some of the worst cases of hungry children could be found in households where the adults seemed relatively well-fed. The weakened toddler whined for impossible things like milk or simply had no desire to eat. In fact, anorexia, or a rejection of food, occurs naturally in malnutrition, often caused by infection or a deficiency of a nutrient like zinc.

Other anthropologists had already linked the slow starvation of the Alto people with the languor, or "laziness," attributed to workers in northern Brazil, as well as to a manic-depressive personality or melancholia. In addition to the physical changes of hunger, Scheper-Hughes observed mood changes: depression, giddiness, irritability, bravado, "followed by uncontrolled weeping; fierce, crazy anger; and the lashing out even at those who would be of assistance. Alternating with rage are passivity and indifference, as if one were absorbed by some distant or interior reality."

In 1985, the anthropologist returned to Alto do Cruzeiro in the first of four more visits. Extreme poverty was still the norm. The hunger of the Alto had not been resolved. Instead, it had been hidden, in this case by a medicalization that transformed the accompanying signs of hunger—shakiness, weakness, fainting, insomnia, anxiety—into a more psychological and subtle illness. Suddenly the people were suffering from *nervos*, or nerves, best treated with tranquilizers, tonics, antidepressants, sleeping pills, painkillers, and vitamins. People commonly visited the medical clinics now, as well as the many new pharmacies, where they could get drugs for free or on credit or even where they bought drugs in place of food. They were now more likely to say, "I couldn't sleep all night and I woke up shaking and crying with *nervos*" than that they went to bed hungry and woke up hungry. Now they fainted from *nervos*. They were irritable from *nervos*.

A sick body reinforced the image that the Alto people had of themselves as weak, flawed, and lacking in some vital force. They were easily convinced that their best hope lay in "the magical efficacy of drugs." Also, in an oppressive political environment where workers had few rights, the metaphor of *nervos* was a safer way to express anger and unhappiness. "I am sick," is a less dangerous statement to make than "I am hungry." Scheper-Hughes wrote, "A hungry body exists as a potent critique of the society in which it exists. A sick body implicates no one. . . . To acknowledge hunger, which is not a disease but a social illness, would be tantamount to political suicide for leaders whose power has come from the same plantation economy that has produced the hunger in the first place."

The social responses to widespread hunger are varied, dependent to some degree on history and culture, on politics, on economics, and on personal choice. Yet these responses are still grounded in the body. Our faces change. Our skin discolors. Our hearts slow. Our bones weaken. And we look at our children differently.

ANOREXIA NERVOSA

IN THEIR TWO VOLUMES ON THE BIOLOGY OF human starvation, the scientists in the Minnesota Experiment briefly discussed anorexia nervosa, a disease in which the patient and famine victim "meet on the common ground of calorie restriction." Since anorectics usually starve in a sanitary environment of flush toilets and medical support, they can survive extreme weight loss. The Minnesota researchers cited a 1947 case in which a 24-year-old woman, at 5' 2", went from 122 to 50 pounds in 18 months. The patient was up and about and reasonably active. She did not remain for treatment. The researchers wrongly believed that the anorexic woman was indifferent to eating and defined anorexia nervosa as the loss of desire for food in the absence of an organic reason for this loss. They rightly observed that anorectics often showed a manic behavior that contrasted with the apathy normally seen in starvation.

As early as the seventeenth century, doctors looked at these hungry women and saw disease rather than choice. The observer of one fasting maid in 1669 speculated that her condition was due to ferment in the blood related to ovulation. It was a diagnostic shift, from the miraculous world of Catherine of Siena, *anorexia mirabilis,* to the self-destruction of Karen Carpenter, anorexia nervosa. That shift should not equate the two. Historians caution that the experiences of these two women are not to be confused one for the other. As society changed, as the lives of women changed, voluntary starvation became a different phenomenon. What exactly that phenomenon is eludes us. In 1889, Sigmund Freud wrote that the "well known anorexia of young girls seems to be a melancholia occurring where sexuality is undeveloped." Later, doctors thought the disease might be a dysfunction of the pituitary or thyroid. That theory was proved wrong, as was the next, which proposed a fixation on pregnancy. The fasting maid is no longer a miracle. She is still a mystery.

In the past fifty years, anorexia nervosa has gone from rare to seemingly common. Most of us know of a friend of a friend, or someone even closer. We all know about the celebrities, especially the ones that died. Therapists report that more patients seem to be taking their cues from the media. Inadvertently, stories about anorexia nervosa promote anorexia nervosa. Meanwhile, the Internet is reaching a new audience with pro-anorexia websites that share tips on how to self-starve. According to the National Association of Anorexia Nervosa and Associated Disorders, one in one hundred adolescent females in the United States is anorectic. Men are less vulnerable, possibly because more women desire to be "small" and so more women diet, a major trigger for an eating disorder. The condition can be found in most ethnic groups and economic classes and in countries from Sweden to Australia. It is not confined to adolescents. Older adults are beginning to self-starve, especially women facing middle age.

The medical criteria for defining anorexia nervosa are a refusal to eat and maintain a normal weight, an intense fear of gaining weight, a disturbed body image—the patient feels fat—and a loss of over 15 percent of normal weight. Females have three or more consecutively missed periods. Anorectics are often described as perfectionist, dependant, and introverted. Emotionally, they suffer from depression, low self-esteem, and mood swings. Physically, prolonged malnutrition can damage the heart, kidney, stomach, and liver. Perhaps 6–10 percent of serious cases die, the highest rate for any mental illness. (One twenty-one-year study puts that rate at over 15 percent, including deaths by suicide.) As well as a general breakdown of the body, anorectics are vulnerable to sudden death, probably from heart arrhythmia. Recovery takes years, and about 50 percent, even with treatment, make only partial or no recovery. They become isolated from their family and friends. They need frequent medical attention. Their life constricts to the number of calories in an orange, the number on a scale. It is not only the body, not only the heart, that gets smaller.

Genes play a role. Eating disorders run in families, and identical twins are more likely both to have eating disorders than fraternal twins. Genes for personality traits such as obsessive-compulsive behavior may be part of the necessary psychological framework. Since the disease often begins with adolescence, scientists are looking at the triggers for hormone production. Too high or too low levels of brain chemicals also affect how an individual responds to hunger and weight loss. Other systems might be involved. A dysfunctional response to stress could produce a chronic aroused state that suppresses appetite even as it explains the hyperactivity of anorectics. In the 1990s, Dr. Hans

Hoek from the Hague Psychiatric Institute spent three years looking for medical records of anorexia nervosa on Curaçao, a Caribbean island where people still thought body fat was beautiful. He found cases proportional to the number in European populations. His view on eating disorders shifted from the social-cultural to the neural-biological.

Still, no one discounts culture. "Genes load the gun," explained one pamphlet on anorexia nervosa. "Environment pulls the trigger." The earlier saints and fasting maids mirrored contemporary ideas about women and God and food. Today, the alignment of female beauty with thinness has been promoted through a fantasy/reality created in movies, television, and magazine photos. The achievement of thinness through dieting is a multi-billion-dollar industry that has been gathering speed for over a hundred years; all the power of capitalism focused on convincing you that you need to lose weight. The influence of the media is highlighted in places like Fiji, where a hefty body was once considered attractive. In the 1990s, the introduction of Western television coincided with a serious rise in eating disorders among adolescent girls.

Social ideas about thinness or body image might lead women into a pattern of dieting. Something else turns a pattern into a prison. It could be a physical predisposition. It could be family dynamics, an adolescent response to overprotective or controlling parents. It could be a response to adolescence itself, a fear of becoming an adult. It could be sexual abuse or childhood trauma. If a young woman desires control in her life, for whatever reason, anorexia nervosa will narrow her world to one important activity in her control.

Voluntary starvation is further complicated by its involuntary effects. The biology of hunger may account for some or much of the symptoms of anorectics, and the biology of recovery may account for their high relapse.

Fifty years after the Minnesota Experiment, psychiatrist Elke Eckert returned to look at the original data. She also tracked down and interviewed nineteen surviving subjects, all of whom had gone on to become college graduates, six with doctorates and one with a master's. Of the original thirty-six men, eleven had died and six could not be found, including the four who had left the experiment early.

During semi-starvation, the Minnesota volunteers developed many of the traits of an anorectic. They became depressed. They had low self-esteem. They withdrew socially. They had little interest in sex. They compulsively hoarded things. They played with their food, creating rituals that extended a meal for hours.

In Jennifer Shute's novel *Life Size*, the anorectic character eats mathematically, "Slowly, delicately, precisely, I cut the piece of toast into halves, then quarters, then eighths, then sixteenths, and daintily convey each piece to my mouth, allowing three minutes between bites. Then, in the same way, I eat exactly half the slice of cantaloupe."

Like anorectics, the Minnesota volunteers became obsessed with all aspects of food. They changed their career plans and dreamed of becoming cooks. "To say that I 'lost' my appetite during those years would be a joke," Caroline Knapp wrote in her memoir of anorexia nervosa. "On the contrary, I ate, slept, and breathed appetite. I thought about food constantly, pored over food magazines, and restaurant reviews like a teenage boy with a pile of porn."

In later interviews, the Minnesota subjects remembered how staff and researchers at the laboratory began to look fat to them.

The men were painfully aware of their own emaciation. And yet, the thick flesh of a doctor's arm, his solid cheeks, those rolls of skin bulging at the neck . . . was that really normal?

The anorectic patient of one psychiatrist, Hilda Bruche, looks into a mirror and briefly sees that she is too skinny. "But I can't hold onto it. I feel inwardly that I am larger than that—no matter what I tell myself. Even last summer I felt large, that was when I was at my lowest, sixty-seven pounds, but I felt I was very large."

The delusional world of the anorectic can seem extreme. Yet four of the thirty-six volunteers in the Minnesota Experiment had extreme reactions to semi-starvation, ranging from neurosis to a psychotic breakdown. They wept. They broke things. They contemplated suicide. A man cut off his fingers. These had been healthy, strong-minded, conscientious objectors, screened for their physical and mental well-being. Hunger drove them a little crazy.

Elke Eckert also looked at the refeeding stage of the Minnesota Experiment. Once off a restricted diet, the Minnesota volunteers tended to binge, gobbling five to six thousand calories at a sitting. The men felt they had little control over their eating and would gorge themselves to the point of distress, until they vomited or—in one case—had to be hospitalized for heart failure. Their hunger was outside their will, like the "alien force" some anorectics describe when they sneak to the refrigerator late at night, stuffing food into their mouths, first the leftover spaghetti, then a bowl of cereal, then half a loaf of bread.

The men also became overweight. The Minnesota researchers examined six men eight months after the end of semi-starvation and found they had an average of 39 percent more fat than they had had entering the experiment. Eckert determined that her nineteen men eventually gained an average of 18 percent of their original weight. The extreme example was the genial Jim Graham, who would put on a hundred pounds and stay heavy for three years.

Moreover, the new fat had a new distribution. "It certainly wasn't in the same place," one man remembered. Studies confirm that when anorectics gain weight, most of that is in fat mass, with most of the fat accumulating in the trunk area, around their waist and hips. This happens even when the patient is still underweight, still painfully thin, but now with a pot belly. The less trunk fat the woman had to begin with, the more she gains in that area.

The physical recovery from starvation includes the very things anorectics fear the most: the uncontrollable power of hunger and excess fat. Eckert wonders if this isn't why so many anorectics become bulimics, vomiting up what they have just eaten, frantic with the success of their therapy.

In other ways, anorexia feeds on itself. In malnutrition, a true loss of appetite is a protective strategy that prevents the body from the stress of too much food too soon. Malnourished people can also lose their appetite because of a nutrient deficiency or hidden infection. Hunger is often blunted in complete fasting, and some anorectics approach that, eating only a few hundred calories a day. For the malnourished, eating also becomes associated with discomfort, as refeeding did for the Minnesota men with their complaints of stomach pain and bloating. An addiction to starvation may be partially fueled by what the body perceives as good.

Still, the anorectic and the "normally" starving man or woman have physical differences. At the University of Minnesota, in the twenty-fourth week of semi-starvation, the conscientious objectors sprawled on their beds and slumped in their chairs. Anorectics would be doing jumping jacks. They would have welcomed the treadmill tests. Although the high energy of these young women may be connected to their desire to burn calories, Elke Eckert sees the constant jiggling and hyperactivity as part of a compulsion to move. The starving man increases his food-seeking activity and decreases all others; the anorectic does the opposite.

There are other oddities. Levels of chemicals that signal satiety for food are often high in anorectics, not low. However, signals for hunger like ghrelin are also high, so that anorectics may be getting conflicting messages.

Psychiatrist Shan Guisinger developed the Adapted to Flee Famine Hypothesis to explain these differences. Guisinger theorized that most of the symptoms of anorexia nervosa are a result of weight loss, not a cause, and that these symptoms were once adaptive, a holdover from when foragers had to migrate away from famine. People who inherited this response to low body-weight—an inclination to stop eating and start traveling, accompanied by increased energy—were more likely to survive times of food shortage. Guisinger pointed out that anorexia nervosa can develop whenever a person loses weight, either fasting for politics (two female Irish Republican Army hunger strikers went on to die of anorexia nervosa) or for religious reasons (Catherine of Siena and others) or for beauty or control (the case of many women today). Culture might account for some aspects of the modern disease—the anorectic's intense fear of getting fat or the role of family dynamics. The biology of perfectionism might help people persist in dieting. But whatever the cause for weight loss, those individuals with the inherited adaptive response to famine are now vulnerable to its maladaptation.

Perhaps significantly, forms of anorexia nervosa also occur in animals. Particularly in adolescence, certain breeds of lean pigs are susceptible to a wasting anorexia accompanied by restlessness. Rats become hyperactive when starved, female rats sooner than male. Given an activity wheel, rats restricted in food will run until they die.

It is one more theory, in a subject open to discussion. People who know this disease well do not speak with too much certainty. The causes of anorexia nervosa are not only multiple; they interact with each other. Culture reinforces genes. Biology spins experience. The complexity of one woman's self-starvation might yet be a mix of chemistry, *Vogue,* Father's expectations, and ancient imperatives.

. . .

Like obesity, the rise of anorexia nervosa has generated new research in hunger and its effects. How do we deal with osteoporosis in a twenty-year-old? What is the role of electrolytes in semi-starvation? At the National Institutes of Health, Angelo Del Parigi would like to do PET scans of anorectic and bulimic patients. What is going on in the anorectic's brain? Where does her energy come from?

We have learned new ways of talking about hunger, thinking about hunger, analyzing hunger. Some of them are old ways. Philosopher Susan Bordo wrote of a dualism between mind and body in which the body is not self, "fastened and glued" to me, "nailed" and "riveted" to me—just as Plato described it a long time ago. Similarly, for Descartes and Augustine, the body was a swamp, a cage, a fog, and an enemy. The anorectic understands the language of dualism very well. She may refer to herself as a prisoner who wants to get out of the body. She may want to be rid of the body altogether.

The religious impulse toward asceticism also cannot be denied. In Michelle Mary Lelwica's *Starving for Salvation*, an anorectic described her jutting ribs and concave stomach, "I don't know where my intestines go, where my liver flees, what can be left between skin and spine. It's so spare I believe I can push right through, touching bones, muscles, my structural essence . . . oddly I feel as though I've been cleansed. I wonder idly if sacrifice is at the heart of my life."

Some feminists see oppression in this disease: the struggle of women finding their place in a man's world. Although the anorectic has been socialized to suppress her needs, she finds she can not, and so she tries to control them. In this view, anorexia nervosa is a means of expression, a protest, and a hunger strike. The problem is patriarchy; self-starvation is a particularly bad solution.

Some analysts believe that modern images of boyish slimness are a rejection of traditional female values connected to menstruation, pregnancy, childbirth, and lactation. The anorectic has sentenced herself to live out this rejection, to deny her round, womanly body. In return, the culture of beauty, the culture of youth, the culture of perfection offers her—what?

Some anorectics understand their disease best as a personal metaphor. Caroline Knapp remembered her puzzlement when a therapist asked how she had fun. What was her "appetite" for life? What did she hunger for and desire? Her anorexia "elevated to an art form" what she understood appetite to be about: "Weighing, measuring, calculating, monitoring. Withholding and then overcompensating."

Some explanations are more prosaic. An anorectic tells a BBC interviewer that the reasons she wanted to eat less and lose weight weren't about body image or fashion. "It was more that I started a diet and it sort of filled a gap in my life, it almost fulfilled a purpose and became, it became my way of coping with life and the difficulties I was having. It was almost like a screen that I could hide behind. It meant that I didn't need other people, I just had anorexia and anorexia became my best friend."

HUNGRY CHILDREN

ONE MORE WORLD WAR II STORY. IN 1940, the Germans occupied the Netherlands, a small, densely populated country dependent on the importation of food. By July 1944, the average daily ration per adult was 1,350 calories. That September, allied forces entered the Netherlands and advanced toward the Rhine. To support their efforts, the Dutch government-in-exile in London called for a general railroad strike, and Dutch workers responded by stopping rail traffic. The Germans punished the region with an embargo on food transport. By mid-November, the allies had liberated parts of the Netherlands but were unable to reach six major western cities. Under the embargo, a chronic food shortage turned into famine. From October 1944 to May 1945, through what the Dutch would call the Hunger Winter, people began to starve.

The first cases of edema were admitted to the hospitals in January 1945. One medical officer reported that not much relief could be offered these patients. By February, special "starvation hospitals" were giving people who had lost 25 percent of their weight some extra rations. But not everyone could reach these hospitals in time, and many died at home or on the street. The last four weeks before liberation were the worst, with people eating as little as five hundred calories a day.

The Dutch are good record keepers. When the Germans occupied the Netherlands, they found the Jewish population labeled and documented (as were the Catholics and Protestants), easy to find, easy to gather for shipment to the camps. The same efficient record keeping helped a group of scientists in the late 1960s who wanted to study the effects of starvation on children—specifically on fetal development. They were able to look at hundreds of thousands of hospital records for men conceived and born during the Hunger Winter and to follow these men through the physical and psychological tests done later by the Dutch military on all eighteen-year-olds.

The researchers entered the study with a hypothesis. They predicted that prenatal exposure to famine would result in mental deficiencies in adult survivors. Famine babies would be less smart.

As expected, there were fewer births, only a third of the normal rate, reflecting the infertility associated with hunger. Of the babies born, more than usual died. The idea that a pregnant woman's resources are used to sustain her fetus is only partially true. The mother absorbs the first impact of food shortage. But at a certain point, if she is not getting enough nutrition, her survival outranks that of the child. In the Dutch study, starvation in the first trimester caused an increase in abnormal development of the fetus's central nervous system, premature birth, still births, and death in the first three months of life. The fetus in the second trimester seemed more protected but became vulnerable again in the third trimester, with a higher risk of low birth weight and death in the first months. Infant deaths at 7–29 days went from fewer than 4 per 1,000 births in a normal year to 22 per 1,000 births in the Hunger Winter. The average length of the baby and the baby's head circumference also declined, although not as much as weight.

Among surviving adult men, the researchers found more spina bifida, hydrocephalus, and cerebral palsy. (Partly as a result of this study, pregnant women are advised to take folate supplements to prevent neural tube defects.) The researchers did not find that survivors conceived or born during the famine months were less intelligent or mentally competent than other populations. Either those infants with brain damage had already died or the brain, again, was showing its resilience to starvation.

Scientists keep returning to the Dutch Hunger Winter. In the 1970s, they looked for signs of obesity in the records of three hundred thousand nineteen-year-old military draftees who had been exposed to famine in utero. Men who had been exposed in the first half of gestation were fatter than non-exposed men. Those who had been exposed in the second half of gestation were less fat than non-exposed men. Another study done in the 1990s on seven hundred subjects in their fifties showed that women who had been exposed to famine in utero in early gestation had higher body weight and waist circumference than non-exposed women. Both men and women exposed in early gestation had higher cholesterol levels, with less of the good cholesterol that protects the circulatory system. Adults exposed in mid- to late-gestation had a less efficient metabolization of carbohydrates. In other studies, prenatal malnutrition increased the risk of mental illness. Famine in early gestation meant more cases of schizophrenia, schizoid/schizotypal personality disorder, and paranoid states. Famine in later gestation resulted in more psychoses, such as bipolar disorder.

In short, the fetus's response to hunger affects an adult throughout his or her life. Those changes may be as subtle as a larger dress size or as blatant as madness.

. . .

Children conceived or born during the Dutch Hunger Winter experienced a starvation that lasted five months or less, followed by a lifetime of normal nutrition. For most hungry children, however, malnutrition is long-term. Remarkably, how long-term malnutrition affects a child has taken us over a century to understand.

In 1858, at a fund-raiser speech for the Hospital of Sick Children, novelist Charles Dickens spoke of his recent visit to the city of Edinburgh: "There lay, in an old egg box, which the mother had begged from a shop, a little, feeble, wasted, wan, sick child. With his little wasted face and his little hot worn hands folded over his breast, and his little bright eyes looking steadily at us." Dickens was describing the condition of marasmus, from the Greek *marasmos*, a wasting away. The term is still used for starving infants and children who appear shrunken or wizened, their weight 60 percent or less of what would be expected for their age. In a marasmic child, the rib outline shows clearly, and there is no fat on the arms, legs, shoulders, buttocks, and thighs so that the skin hangs in loose folds. Atrophy of the gut and microbial disease commonly cause diarrhea. The child may seem hyperalert, the eyes very bright.

In the nineteenth and early twentieth century, marasmus and related infections were a common cause of death among poor children everywhere. In 1915, in eleven orphanages in New York, 422 children in 1,000 died, compared to a city-wide number of 87 in 1,000. Today, we see marasmus mostly in the developing countries of Asia, Africa, the Middle East, and South and Central America. The background is often famine, usually associated with war.

In 1935, pediatrician Cicely Williams recorded for the medical journal *The Lancet* the clinical details of another form of childhood malnutrition. In the language of the Gold Coast of Africa, kwashiorkor means "disease of the displaced child." A new baby takes the mother's breast and the older sibling, usually one or two years of age, is weaned onto an inadequate diet of gruel or porridge. What one researcher called "the florid nature of the symptoms" includes edema, sores of the mucus membranes, skin lesions that look like burns, peeling skin, diarrhea, and irritability. Dark hair may lighten and turn blonde or reddish. The stomach protrudes due to gas and bacteria in the small bowel. Steroid hormones are not being fully eliminated, causing feminization like rounding of the face and long eyelashes. Growth is retarded, even before other symptoms appear. While children with the wasting signs of marasmus usually respond quickly to extra food, children with kwashiorkor may not.

In field reports spanning seventy years, different researchers described the same psychological effects. Children with kwashiorkor are bad tempered and easily upset, when they are not dull and listless. They have no interest in their surroundings, not even toys or other children. According to a paper from 1956, these children "wake easily and then react in a hostile way, weeping and distressed." They have long monotonous cries. They lie or sit for hours without moving, their faces a mask. They often refuse food. Medical attention is resented with an intensity "unexpected in its violence." Often the doctor or researcher is surprised at the "quality of hopelessness and despair that is characteristic of kwashiorkor" when compared to other serious illnesses.

Kwashiorkor had been seen earlier in children fed poor and monotonous diets, what doctors then called the "flour-feeding injury of Europe" and "the swelling disease of Vietnam." Once the disease had an official name, it was found everywhere in the world. While marasmus could be seen as a lack of energy—not enough calories to sustain life—kwashiorkor seemed to be caused by a more specific lack of protein. These children usually had low concentrations of protein in their plasma and responded best to a diet that included milk. Also, the disease was more prevalent in countries where the staple diet was low in protein, such as rice, cassava roots, or low-quality maize. In the 1950s, the World Health Organization concluded that kwashiorkor was our most serious nutritional disorder and fixed on protein deficiency as the problem to solve. Milk was a good food for recovery but milk was not always available. Into the 1970s, nutritionists focused on the development of high-protein foods for weaning.

Meanwhile, most malnourished children continued to die from marasmus, not enough food to eat. Slowly, policy makers realized that this was the more common cause of death. Diets without adequate protein were actually rare; diets without enough calories were not. People also began to look at other problems in child malnutrition, deficiencies in iron, Vitamin A, and iodine that were causing widespread anemia, blindness, and retardation. At the same time, new research raised doubts about the relationship of kwashiorkor to protein. In fact, high-protein diets did not seem to be working very well. Children with severe malnutrition went into hospitals, were supervised and fed, and still died at the rate of 20–40 percent. Sometimes the rate was higher. A few scientists became interested in the role of micronutrients. Significantly, patients suffering from a disease that blocks the absorption of zinc have many of the same symptoms as malnutrition. In an Indonesian study, Vitamin A supplements reduced the deaths of malnourished preschoolers by 34 percent. What did that mean?

In 1980, experiments at Jamaica's Tropical Research Metabolism Unit showed that children with kwashiorkor actually did better when fed a low-protein diet, one even lower in protein than what they had received before admission to the unit. Mike Golden, a nutritionist in these experiments, suspected that the more florid symptoms of kwashiorkor were caused by oxidative stress—an imbalance that occurs when free radicals damage too many cells. Further research suggested that oxidative stress is triggered in malnourished children by infection. The body defends against infection or toxins by producing free radicals to help kill the invading organisms. Later, the body must deal with these free radicals, using vitamins and trace metals, which serve as antioxidants and protect against free radical damage. But children with kwashiorkor are deficient in these micronutrients, partly from a poor diet, partly because infection itself can cause a loss of micronutrients. In addition, these children frequently have excess iron, which can generate more free radicals.

A case of measles, then, might precipitate the symptoms of kwashiorkor. Microbial infection in the small bowel also seems to initiate the disease, as might toxins like bacteria or fungi in food or the environment. (The low plasma protein in a child with kwashiorkor is probably also due to infection in the body, which causes the liver to stop synthesizing certain kinds of measurable protein in favor of other compounds that repair cells and tissue damage.)

Golden divided nutrients into Type I and Type II. Type I nutrients are normally stored in the body but have been depleted in malnutrition. They include antioxidants like Vitamins A, C, E, and beta-carotene, riboflavin, thiamine, nicotinic acid, and selenium. Type II, or "growth," nutrients are not stored in the body and must be consumed on a regular basis. They include essential amino acids (which are, to some extent, stored in protein), sulfur, zinc, phosphorous, and potassium. While a diet low in protein does not lead to kwashiorkor, it does result in stunting or wasting, as does a deficiency in Type II nutrients.

Throughout this research, for over forty years after World War II, children with severe malnutrition kept dying, even with medical care. Mike Golden believes that this high mortality rate resulted from the world's insistence on protein deficiency as the cause of kwashiorkor. Children were being refed with a high-protein diet that stressed their already abnormal metabolism. In fact, he says, kwashiorkor is caused by the lack of "a series of micronutrients that protect us against oxidation, against going rancid."

Children with edema were also being falsely diagnosed as dehydrated. These children were given salt when the cells in their body had excess salt due to the malfunction of the cell's pumping mechanisms. They were given diuretics that led to potassium loss in their urine when their cells were dangerously low in potassium. When potassium was given as a supplement, it was sometimes given too quickly. Iron was also given too soon, increasing free radical damage. Many of these mistakes ended in heart failure, mistakenly seen as pneumonia.

In the 1990s, Mike Golden helped develop a series of therapeutic foods that tried to include all the nutrients needed to treat
childhood malnutrition, in the right amount, in the right order.
Phase I milk, or F75, is for the initial recovery from severe malnutrition. With its balance of electrolytes, vitamins, and minerals
added to dried skim milk, sugar, and vegetable oil, the diet is essentially a drug for an abnormal metabolism. Phase II milk, or
F100, is designed to maximize weight gain without stressing the
child's system. Later, a porridge called SP450 helps a child put on
weight quickly and is suitable for all ages. First produced com-
mercially, these formulas are now in the public domain.

Scientists have reached the agreement that before weight gain
or tissue growth, before the body can handle excess energy, the
balance of nutrients has to be restored. This does not contradict
the findings of the Minnesota Experiment so much as supplement them. Hunger takes many forms and is more complex than
we imagined. In truth, we still do not fully understand what
causes kwashiorkor. We do not fully understand the mechanisms
of edema or the role of micronutrients. We do not know yet the
best strategy for treating severely malnourished children. We
have just learned what not to give them.

Around the world, eleven children die every minute from
hunger, even if the official report reads measles or diarrhea or
malaria. One hundred and fifty million children are underweight.
One hundred and eighty-two million children are stunted. While
the percentage of hungry children has declined in the last thirty
years, their number still seems impossibly huge.

. . .

In 1984, a BBC film about a famine in Ethiopia opened with a crowd of shrouded, motionless figures. Suddenly, viewers saw a baby, the typical too-tiny body and too-large head, the eyes closed, the mouth open in a despairing cry. A mother cuddled the child close to her face. The camera moved to the child's swollen knees, his head again, his gaze flickering past, his gaze meeting yours. *He sees you. He knows you.* Next, there was another child. This one was dead, carried in a parent's arms. Now, a three-year-old actually died in front of the camera, on her mother's lap. Perhaps 470 million people would watch this death.

In the history of food aid, the BBC film was a turning point for the images it used and the numbers it reached. Save the Children, one of the few aid organizations in Ethiopia at the time, received 1.4 million dollars in donations in one month, the Catholic Relief Services almost 3 million dollars. Later, the celebrities of Live Aid and Band Aid got the attention of groups who had never thought much about developing countries before. Twenty million people participated in a six-mile run in 274 cities in 78 countries. "We Are the World" was the movement's slogan, and that is what those pictures had done, if only briefly: they had bridged the gap between self and world.

Less than a decade later, the media again highlighted graphic scenes of starvation, this time of a famine in Somalia. A journalist for *USA Today* described a blind three-year-old girl crouching beside her emaciated mother. As they lay on the ground, the child groped for her mother's mouth and tried to feed her. "You can take my food," the girl said, as she combed her mother's hair with her hand. "But it was too late," the reporter wrote. "The mother was dead. And no one had the heart to tell the child." *Time Magazine* highlighted one of its stories with the photo of a baby, its eyes glued shut by flies, sucking on a limp rag. Then you looked closer and understood. The rag was a breast. These images eventually inspired the American government to military action, and in December 1992, it sent over 20,000 marines to Somalia to guard ports and food shipments.

In *Compassion Fatigue*, journalist Susan Moeller explains why children are so prevalent in stories and photographs of starvation. Children are not yet linked to prejudices of skin color or culture or politics. Instead, starving children "create an imperative statement" and "bring moral clarity to the complex story of a famine."

At the same time, the icon of children in famine is a Western bias. In many of the places where extreme hunger exists, the survival of adults might be viewed as more important. Famine does not simply affect individuals; it can destroy societies. And the future of a group does not lie in its orphaned babies but in those men and women who can go on to reproduce again. In famine, a focus on women and children highlights biology: here is a mother who cannot feed her child, a breakdown in the natural order of life. This focus obscures who and what is to blame for the famine, politically and economically, and can lead to the belief that a biological response, more food, will solve the problem.

The marines learned that when they went to Somalia. Without a larger context, the images of starving children did not prepare Americans for the reality of that particular famine—a social and civil struggle that we did not understand and were not willing to remedy. Another image of a dead marine being dragged through the streets of Mogadishu caused Americans to withdraw from Somalia the next fall, leaving a people still hungry and a country still at war.

We do not always know what to do about the pictures we take of hungry children. Susan Moeller tells the story of Kevin Carter, who in 1993 went into yet anther famine area in the Sudan. In the village of Ayod, where twenty people were dying every hour, he worked as a photojournalist until he was exhausted and over-whelmed. Then he wandered away from the feeding centers into the open bush, where he saw an emaciated child collapsed from hunger. He began to photograph her. A vulture landed nearby. After Carter snapped several pictures, "he chased the bird away and watched as the little girl resumed her struggle. Afterward, he said, he sat by a tree, talked to God, cried, and thought about his own daughter Megan."

Kevin Carter's photograph of the vulture and the girl was praised and criticized and won a Pulitzer Prize. When people wondered why he hadn't helped the little girl in some way, he found it difficult to explain that at the time she had been one of hundreds of people starving all around him. Within a year, he committed suicide, saying to a friend, "I'm really, really sorry I didn't pick that child up."

. . .

When an adult is hungry, it happens in the present tense. When a child starves, there is another dimension. It also happens in the future. For a child is potential, in the act of becoming.

Prolonged malnutrition in childhood usually results in a stunt-ing of physical growth. Adults in countries with chronic food shortages are often smaller and shorter than in other countries, and for a time nutritionists wondered if that was a bad thing. Per-haps short stature was an adaptation to hunger. We now think no.

For the child who is not reaching her potential for growth, stunting serves as shorthand for other problems—in organ development, hormonal function, and the immune system. In some cases, stunting can be reversed with enough of the right kind of food before puberty. For most malnourished children, this kind of care will never happen.

To a large degree, however, we do not situate our capacity, our humanness, in the body or in measurements of height and weight, but in the mind. And so, like the researchers of the Dutch Hunger Winter, we return anxiously to how hunger affects cognition, by which we mean how we interact with the world, how we think and engage and create—by which we mean, really, who we are.

From birth to age two, a child's brain grows to 80 percent of its adult size. Scientists used to think that any lack of food at this critical time would cause permanent damage. We saw this in the brains of malnourished rats: a reduction in their cerebral cortex and changes in the brain cells. Later, more research showed that many of these changes could be reversed. Moreover, brain growth in malnourished children can be delayed or put on hold until the age of three and perhaps longer.

For eight years in the 1970s, children in four Guatemalan villages were given one of two supplements: a sweet, thick, high-protein drink called Atole, fortified with vitamins and minerals, or a sweet, clear, fruit-flavored drink called Fresco, also fortified with vitamins and minerals but without protein and with only a third of Atole's calories. The researchers were interested in the effects of added protein. More than two thousand children received the supplements, and every child's health improved in some way. In every village, infant mortality went down. But for the children given the higher-caloric Atole, it went down 69 percent. For the children given the less-nutritious Fresco, it went down 24 percent. Atole improved growth rates in children under three, while children drinking Fresco showed little benefit. Adolescents who had been given Atole in their early years were also taller, heavier, with greater bone density and bone mineral content. The study was a confirmation of good sense: more calories meant more growth and more health.

Over ten years later, a new group of scientists returned to the Guatemalan villages to see what had happened to these children mentally. Some 70 percent of the original participants agreed to help by taking intelligence and academic tests. They ranged in age from eleven to twenty-seven. One study focused on almost seven hundred children who had received the supplements in the prenatal period up to age two, the essential first years. The lucky ones who had received Atole rather than Fresco now did better on tests of intellectual ability, memory, attention span, and general knowledge. Even those at the lowest end of the economic scale did as well as the more privileged children in the village (though not as well as middle-class children from elsewhere in Guatemala), prompting the researchers to describe Atole as "a social equalizer." The children who had Atole during their school years seemed to have taken better advantage of that education; their vocabulary skills were well above those who had received fewer calories.

Other studies from Barbados showed that children with early malnutrition have a higher rate of attention deficit disorder, as well as a significant drop in IQ compared to the control groups. Scientists now think that any extended malnutrition in childhood will affect a child's mental ability in some way. It will change who he or she is in the world.

The researchers in Guatemala did not relate the differences they saw only to nutrition. The development of the human mind is not just an interior process. When children who must conserve energy withdraw from the world, the world withdraws from them. Mothers become less responsive to their less responsive infants. Bonding and emotional attachment may be affected. The malnourished child sits later, crawls later, and walks later. He is less interested in exploring his environment. He doesn't play as much. He is smaller and seen by adults as younger than he is. They expect less of him. They talk to him less. In school, he is less social and active. He is less motivated. His teachers are less interested in him.

In a study on stunted Jamaican children between nine and twenty-four months of age, food supplements alone increased the children's intellectual development. Stimulation or play therapy alone also helped. The best result was when you put the two things together.

A healthy home environment, which can range from a grandmother's presence to access to clean water, can buffer the effects of malnutrition. Equally, as the Guatemalan study showed, good nutrition can buffer the effects of environment; the poor children supplemented with Atole did as well as the more prosperous children of the village, while those children given fewer calories did not.

In a country as rich as the United States, millions of children still suffer from mild to moderate malnutrition that is not buffered by the home. Many of these children are homeless. When they come to school hungry, they have difficulty concentrating. Math problems don't seem very important. They are irritable or apathetic with their peers. Although school breakfast programs are federally funded, over half of American school districts do not have them, and so the children wait for lunch to eat. Children who are mildly malnourished usually have other health problems. In one study of four hundred children in Worcester, Massachusetts, those who regularly experienced hunger (based on interviews and surveys with parents) had high levels of chronic illness, depression, and anxiety. In America, as elsewhere, these problems do not just concern us now. They will also concern us later, when these children are adults.

. . .

According to the 2001 World Health Organization manual, this is how you care for a malnourished child: Weigh the baby and check if her weight is under 70 percent of the standard weight for height. (Remember that an underweight child may only be stunted and not need your immediate attention.) Check if she shows signs of wasting, such as a visible rib outline or hanging skin in the shoulders, arms, buttocks, or thighs. Check if she has edema in both feet. If you see any one of these things, diagnose her as having severe malnutrition. Fortunately, you do not have to distinguish between kwashiorkor or marasmus or marasmic kwashiorkor since the treatment is the same for all.

Take a history and examine the baby for dehydration or shock. You can assume that children with watery diarrhea have some dehydration. But be careful. Dehydration tends to be over-diagnosed. If it seems necessary, rehydrate with an oral solution. Do not use an IV since these solutions often have high sodium and low potassium content. Be alert for over-hydration, which can cause heart failure. If the child's breathing gets faster or if her pulse rate increases, stop rehydration immediately.

Check for low blood sugar. You can assume that any severely malnourished child has hypoglycemia. Give her a solution with 10 percent glucose or sucrose by mouth or through a tube in the nose, followed by the first feeding. This first feeding should start immediately, be appropriate to the child's weight, and continue every two hours, day and night. If possible, divide the first feeding into four and give it every half hour. If you are lucky, you'll be using a milk-based formula that contains just the right amount of protein, carbohydrates, and fat, as well as micronutrients. Don't overfeed.

Check for hypothermia. If the body temperature is below 95°F, start warming the child with blankets, bare skin, a heater, or a lamp.

Check the eyes for Vitamin A deficiency such as spots on the cornea or ulcerations. Give the appropriate drops, and cover her eyes with a pad and bandage. These children may be photophobic and will keep their eyes tightly closed against the light. Be very gentle so as to prevent corneal rupture.

Check for severe anemia. Give a blood transfusion if necessary. (Mike Golden, who helped write the WHO manual, believes it needs to be further revised. The new instructions would emphasize that blood transfusions should be strictly limited. They would also insist, more strongly, that dehydration is overdiagnosed, that any severely malnourished child should be given sugar water rather than any solution with salt, and that protocol needs to be adapted to local conditions, such as a hot desert climate.)

Check for infection and start a course of antibiotics. You don't have to think about this either. You can assume that a malnourished child, even without a fever, has some infection somewhere. Specifically check for signs of meningitis, pneumonia, malaria, tuberculosis, and HIV.

Check for skin problems. The baby may look badly sunburned. She may have ulcerations spreading over her legs, thighs, groin, arms, and behind the ears. These will probably clear up with a zinc supplement and ointment.

Do not use diuretics to treat a child with edema. Do not give too much salt. Although anemia is common and potentially dangerous, it is probably not caused by an iron deficiency and may coexist with iron overload. Do not give iron until later.

Do everything you need to do—rehydrate, feed, warm, give antibiotics—as quickly as you can. Monitor carefully. Later, you'll switch to another formula food. Monitor that transition. Later you'll need to think about play therapy. You'll make toys out of thread and wooden spools. You'll smile and chatter and coax and you'll see remarkable changes. You'll see a dawning, the lift of misery, something wonderful.

PROTOCOLS OF FAMINE

People like me stand outside the world of hunger and feel horrified. We wring our hands. What to do? A few people start doing something. In the fall of 1992, Baidoa, Somalia, was the epicenter of a famine that had already killed 75 percent of children under the age of five. Every day in Somalia, perhaps a thousand people died of malnutrition and disease, a quickening of that country's slow-motion disaster—decades of civil war complicated by drought. In October, the Irish group Concern Worldwide opened in Baidoa the first therapeutic feeding center for adults: nine stick shelters with roofs of plastic sheeting and floors of compacted mud.

While supplementary feeding centers give food to the moderately malnourished, therapeutic feeding centers focus on the severely malnourished and provide a specialized diet with twenty-four-hour care. Like most, this center did not have beds, so everyone slept on the hard mud, on another plastic sheet. The nine shelters held about 140 sick people, segregated into groups: new admissions, severe edema, bloody diarrhea, and pulmonary tuberculosis. Most patients also had a relative to care for them. Steve Collins and Marion White were the doctor and nurse in charge, supported by three local nurses and thirty other attendants and cooks. Frances O'Keefe managed all the Concern programs, which included some twenty thousand children. Because of the violence—kidnappings, gun battles, robberies, random attacks—Steve and Marion had to leave the center every night for a safer house on the outskirts of town.

The therapeutic feeding center only accepted cases of gross malnutrition, patients too ill to stand up to be measured and weighed, or patients with severe edema, or patients with a Body Mass Index below 13.5—a 6'0" man, say, weighing 99 pounds. Between October and March, the center's staff admitted 573 people, roughly half male and half female, ages 15–80. The patients were registered, assessed, and given treatment cards that included a course of antibiotics. They began rehabilitation with a high-energy liquid made of dried skim milk, vegetable oil, and sugar, with added salts and glucose. In an atrophied digestive system, this usually causes diarrhea or vomiting, and the milk had to be further diluted with an oral rehydration solution. Soon the patients were eating, theoretically, six to eight meals a day of sweet tea, rice, beans, oil, fortified biscuits, and bananas, a regimen that included about 16 percent of daily energy in protein.

Despite the specialized diet, despite the high staff-to-patient ratio, despite conscientious care, the treatment didn't seem to be working. Almost half the deaths were in the first week. Males with severe edema seemed particularly at risk. "It was really a hospice," Frances O'Keefe will tell me later at a dinner party in Dublin, Ireland, at the home of the director of Concern Worldwide. "People were just coming there to die."

In 1992, Steve Collins knew of the work done by Mike Golden in Jamaica, which suggested that adults with severe malnutrition, as well as children, responded best to a low-protein diet. But no one had field-tested that idea. No one had done any field work with malnourished adults since the end of World War II and the liberation of the concentration camp survivors. In many ways, the Minnesota Experiment remained the final word, and that had been on young men who lost only 24 percent of their body weight, with a Body Mass Index of about 18. In later famines in Africa, malnourished adults with BMIs of 18 seemed to recover with diets that had a protein ratio of 19 percent, and organizations like Concern had adopted that strategy. No one knew what worked best for adults with BMIs of 13 or lower, the Somalians that Steve and Marion were admitting to their center.

The nine stick shelters in Baidoa became the field test. On December 5, Steve offered meals with half the usual protein to eleven men and women with edema who were not showing signs of recovery. The new diet had a higher percentage of fat and would be increasingly diluted to prevent diarrhea. The response was dramatic. People who had refused food began to eat. Their edema diminished. They gained weight. In a few days, the staff knew that to continue the higher protein diet for very ill or edematous patients was unethical. This would not be a controlled study, except in the sense that more people died before December 5, under the high-protein regime, than after December 5, under the low-protein regime. "At that point," Frances remembers, "we became a real therapeutic feeding center, a place to get better."

In 1992, researchers thought that the limit of human survival ended with a BMI of 12. But the Concern center saw patients survive with BMIs as low as 8.7—a 5'8" woman weighing fifty-eight pounds. For adults over 25 with BMIs under 11, the survival rate was 65 percent and an extraordinary 82 percent for young adults, ages 15–24. In part, this may have been due to the Somalians' tall, thin body type, warm climate, and gradual adjustment to food shortage. In part, more Somalians lived because they were fed less protein.

Reducing protein helped only patients with edema. Patients with marasmus seemed unaffected, for good or bad. In all cases, the new diet was more easily available and cost almost half as much, about a dollar a day. In the end, over 72 percent of the people who came to the Concern center lived. They left the center when they had no infectious disease, a good appetite, weight gain, and the ability to care for themselves. They were given a ride back to their village with a discharge packet that included a sheet of plastic, a hoe, a machete, seeds, pots and pans, a blanket, water containers, and some cloth.

The Baidoa research looked briefly at sex differences. Anecdotally, women seem better adapted to famine. The data from the Dutch Hunger Winter suggests that women can survive with lower BMIs than men. In Baidoa, male patients had more severe grades of edema and a worse prognosis for each grade. However, the people who came to the Baidoa center had either walked or been carried by friends and family, and the greater number of males with severe edema might have reflected the greater willingness of people to help males. Similarly, the women who walked to the center could have been self-selected for resilience.

Steve believes that the low-protein diet put less stress on vital organs, especially the liver and kidneys. Many edematous patients show signs of liver failure—jaundice and rashes—while marasmic patients have better liver function. Edematous patients also have a more disordered metabolism, which reacts badly to excess energy, eventually causing heart failure.

The diet was key. But Frances O'Keefe says that other things are equally important, perhaps more important. Adults who have lost the desire to eat have to be so patiently coaxed, nurtured, seduced. There is an inner voice whispering *life,* and they have to listen. Frances remembers how a woman who had lost her family rallied only when an orphan came into the feeding center, someone else she could care for (this was not the center in Baidoa, this was another place, another year, another famine). Frances remembers a young girl, "so thin, so frail, so sick," who, one morning, wanted to have her hair combed. "After that," Frances says, sitting with me on the couch at the home of the director of Concern Worldwide, "after they have made that decision, the ability of the human body to survive is amazing. They may still get diarrhea. They may still get an infection. They will still live."

"The banana man, the banana man! That's what they called Steve!" Frances smiles easily, remembering Baidoa, that heyday time, when people were suddenly living. "But those Somalians, they also love their camel meat, their camel milk. Once in a while, we'd give someone just a little bit, just to get them started. We had to sneak it in."

I must have looked confused, for Frances glances around the party, at this group of a dozen people talking as they balance plates of food. She is searching for Steve Collins, who is also here, in the middle of a joke, laughing with our host. "Oh, well, you know, because of Steve. It wasn't on the diet."

Steve joins us and they both agree: adults are much harder to care for than children, physically and psychologically. Children die faster because of their greater energy needs, but they also recover faster, and a starving child can be "a new kid" within a week. Adults have different nutritional requirements. Adults have more edema. Adults heal slowly. In Baidoa, adults suffered from contracted limbs and lower limb wasting from months of squatting, and they needed lengthy physical therapy. Anorexic adults are particularly difficult: nothing duplicates the authority of a mother feeding her child. Adults hate to feel helpless. They resent being bullied. They don't want to be fed with a spoon. They don't want a feeding tube up their nose. They remember their families. They remember their homes. They remember their dignity. They can die from sorrow.

Perhaps because it is so hard to care for adults, perhaps because of the Western bias toward saving children, Steve also noticed in Baidoa that adults were being remarkably neglected. While malnourished children got two meals a day of milk, biscuits, and fortified porridge, adults went to kitchens where they waited hours for a single plate of rice and beans. "The sheer physical struggle of maintaining a place in line weeded out the weak," Steve says. Few of the adults who came to his center that fall would have survived without special care and food.

Steve is astonished by the lack of research being done on adults, as well as the lack of attention in the field. Information on adolescents, he says, is virtually nonexistent. After Baidoa, he wrote papers on the subject, scolding his colleagues, "Many can be saved with just a small redirection of resources toward adult therapeutic units. In saving adults and adolescents, you are saving those who grow the food, create the wealth, and care for children."

The research done in Baidoa showed that adult therapeutic feeding centers could be successful even in cases of extreme emaciation. In 1992, Steve believed that these centers should be included far more frequently in famine relief programs. Six years later, he would change his mind.

In 1992, in Baidoa, Steve Collins had normal hair. Now at a dinner party in 2004, where Steve is wearing a suit and some women have put on nylon stockings, his dreadlocks make the first impression: wild, plentiful, mischievous. His work in Somalia helped redefine therapeutic feeding around the world. After Baidoa, he didn't need to look for a job in relief organizations. He had proved himself, and he could be himself, a person who disliked having to cut his hair, especially when authority figures told him to cut his hair. "Who ever told you to do that?" I wonder out loud. "It probably started early on," he says.

In 1996, Steve headed an Oxfam team in the village of Vonzula, Liberia. Soldiers in that country's civil war regularly seized the produce of local farmers and villagers, often beating and sometimes killing them. People tried to escape the violence by fleeing into the bush, eating whatever they could find, and slowly dying of hunger. A small village like Vonzula no longer had a health center or school or form of central authority. Its population was mobile, with residents suddenly disappearing and strangers, refugees from other villages, suddenly in their place.

The Oxfam team decided against the distribution of dry goods since that attracted looters and made the recipient a target. Only a few miles from Vonzula, forty people would be murdered after the World Food Program gave out a supply of dry rations. Steve and his team focused instead on "wet feeding," providing a meal on site. They came on Saturday, October 5, and by Tuesday, October 8, had admitted to their therapeutic feeding center 150 severely malnourished people. In a supplemental feeding kitchen, they fed another 375. On Thursday, an influx of refugees from a nearby massacre increased these numbers dramatically. Because of fighting in the area, the team had to drive to the village each day, leave before night, and make sure they left nothing behind. Still, there was good news. Everyone was responding well to a diet of high-energy milk and fortified biscuits. A big part of this success was the absence of diarrheal disease. On that very first day, the village well had tested clean for coliforms. Pressed for time, the Oxfam team decided not to chlorinate the water or boil the milk—especially since the children preferred their drink cold.

The first case of cholera appeared on October 13. The cook at the feeding center sickened by October 15. The team admitted twenty severe cases October 17, stopped their feeding programs, and refocused on cholera prevention and treatment. On October 18, Steve and the others were unable to return to the village, and in the next few days, a number of people died—from cholera, not malnutrition. The feeding center itself had probably been a source of infection. Moreover, the establishment of the center had encouraged people to congregate. Many of these were strangers who drank from parts of a creek known by locals to be contaminated. The needs of the feeding center also reduced the available water supply. The village had not told the Oxfam team about cholera in the area, perhaps because they were afraid the team would leave. More to the point, the initial questioning by Steve had been cursory. Vonzula was an unlucky place, these were unlucky times, and who can blame the aid worker for trusting to what little luck he thought he had found? The water had tested clean.

More often than not, famine and disease come braided together, stronger together. In most famines, infection kills first and kills most often. In 1992, among the severely malnourished people of Baidoa, measles and diarrheal disease were the main causes of death. Severe malnutrition disrupts the body's natural barriers against infection. The intestinal walls become more susceptible to invading bacteria, and breakdown of the skin allows more pathogens to enter the body. Now malnutrition makes it harder for the immune system to launch a defense. It takes energy to repair tissue damage, synthesize antibodies, create and send out white blood cells. Hormonal and metabolic changes can also disrupt the immune response, and symptoms such as fever or enlarged lymph nodes are often absent. Importantly, malnutrition and infection change how the body handles micronutrients. As tissues break down, they release trace elements and other nutrients, which are then lost in urine and stools. The diarrhea accompanying infection means more losses of potassium, magnesium, zinc, and Vitamin A.

Some infectious diseases are particularly linked to food deprivation, others not, and others in-between. In the Warsaw ghetto, a weakening of the respiratory and immune systems was related to tuberculosis. Measles acts synergistically with malnutrition, precipitating the symptoms of kwashiorkor, depressing the immune system, and causing anorexia.

And there are social factors. In the controlled environment of the Minnesota Experiment, the semi-starved volunteers did not show an increase in colds or infections. Anorectics often report a resistance to colds and flu. During World War II, famine in countries like the Netherlands did not result in significant epidemics. The picture of modern famine is very different. When people are displaced and forced to move into new areas, they are introduced to new diseases or strains for which they have no resistance. Problems with sanitation and human waste can mean outbreaks of cholera and bacterial dysentery. A lack of soap and water might encourage skin infections or lice, which spread typhus and typhoid. Overcrowding spreads any infectious disease more quickly.

"That's what I learned in Liberia," Steve Collins says. The physician's motto is do no harm. But bringing people together, at feeding centers and in refugee camps, can be a form of doing harm.

In 1998, a famine in the Sudan displaced hundreds of thousands of people. The refrain was familiar, civil war and drought. To make matters worse, the government of Sudan restricted the movement of humanitarian aid. The military diverted relief grain for its use. Donor funds were grossly inadequate until pictures of starving children began to appear in the Western media. Near the town of Wau, from June to August, Steve estimates that more than one hundred therapeutic feeding centers would have been needed to treat sixteen thousand children and adults suffering from severe malnutrition. Instead, there was one: a single twenty-four-hour unit that could handle, at maximum, four hundred people. That center's response was to maintain a high level of medical care but make admission standards more stringent. For example, only children less than 60 percent of normal weight were admitted instead of the usual less than 70 percent.

Steve worked in the Sudan as a consultant. From these experiences, he developed new ideas about admission criteria—who to admit to your center—and prognosis—who is likely to die without your help. Steve suggested that the conventional use of Body

Mass Index was a poor way to determine whether an adult patient should be allowed into a therapeutic feeding center. Instead, in what the famine world bluntly calls a "Chances Model," Steve proposed the use of three clinical signs—dehydration, grade three pitting edema, and the inability to stand—combined with Measurement of the Upper Arm Circumference or MUAC. Grade three pitting edema is swelling demonstrable up to the knee. Measuring the arm circumference reflects the amount of fat under the skin; anything less than 7.28 inches is considered abnormal and less than 6.29 inches severely malnourished. A MUAC of under 6.29 inches or a MUAC of 6.29–7.28, plus any one of the three clinical signs, would be reasonable criteria for admission to intensive care. Patients without these criteria could be treated with supplemental feeding.

Steve returned to the research from Baidoa to see how well the three clinical signs had predicted death. Each one—dehydration, severe edema, and the inability to stand—was independently associated with mortality. The combination of two, however, predicted death with an accuracy greater than 95 percent. Suddenly, Steve is talking about triage, not admission. In a place like the Sudan in 1998, a relief worker could have used these signs quickly, without any equipment, not to determine if the patient needed the intensive care of a therapeutic feeding center but to determine if the patient would get any care at all, not to diagnose how she should help this patient but whether she *should* help this patient, or whether she should move on. This kind of triage, Steve realized, would have better served the starving Sudanese people of Wau in 1998. Moreover, large feeding programs—with reduced care for individuals— would have helped more people overall.

"That's what I learned in the Sudan," Steve says, and it sounds cold, ironically, because Steve runs hot, intense, excitable, compassionate. When you know firsthand that the most severely malnourished patient can be saved with the right treatment, then triage—by workers in the field or by organizations planning what kind of programs to support—is particularly heartbreaking. Still, there is no turning back. Steve responds to a learning curve by climbing it, and he has moved beyond the clinical model, doing as much as possible for each patient, to the public health model, doing as much as possible for many patients. "Our capacity to treat individuals is not the limiting factor," he says now, "and it is not where our resources should go."

In 1999, Steve formed his own company, Valid International, with the mission to improve the quality and accountability of relief work. Valid International partners with organizations like Concern Worldwide to design and implement practical solutions to famine. Steve urged the adoption of "coverage" as one of the criteria for a successful humanitarian assistance. He attended enough meetings to make his point, so that the statistics of a relief program now reflect all the people it was able to reach, not just the success rate for a small group.

Soon he was working with Concern Worldwide again, in Ethiopia's famine of 2000. He could now list the problems he associated with the therapeutic feeding centers he had once championed: (1) They require too many resources in terms of skilled staff and imported products; (2) They are slow to set up; (3) They can treat only a small number of patients; (4) They undermine local health care, which often disappears as soon as outside help is on the scene; (5) They operate in a "cultural vacuum;" strict protocols mean that a well-run therapeutic feeding center in Somalia looks just like one in Malawi; (6) They encourage people to leave their homes and congregate, increasing the risk of disease and stressing the area's public health system; and (7) For severely malnourished children, they require a mother to leave her family—her work, her farming, and her other children—for as long as thirty days.

Steve and colleague Kate Sadler knew of research from Bangladesh that showed that severely malnourished children treated with a week of inpatient care followed by home management recovered as well as children kept in hospitals. The educational program for mothers also had a ripple effect that benefited other parents in the community. This "hearth method" of home-based care seemed to be working in other countries, too, with successful mothers serving as mentors. By now, a ready-to-use therapeutic food, or RUTF, had been developed. This oil-based paste made of peanut butter, sugar, and dried milk, fortified with vitamins and minerals, could be stored for several months and eaten from the packet—no mixing or cooking, no liquid milk to breed bacteria.

No one, yet, had field-tested this idea for acute malnutrition in emergency relief. Ethiopia became the field test. To serve a population of over two hundred thousand hungry people, Concern Worldwide had already set up a dry feeding program from ten distribution points in government-run health clinics. The government did not want relief agencies to set up new centers. So, as severely malnourished children were identified, the ten distribution points now acted as outpatient centers, with local staff quickly trained to assess children, educate mothers, hand out food, and give oral doses of antibiotics, Vitamin A, folic acid, and rehydration solution. The mothers and children then went home and returned every week for a medical checkup, a supply of RUTF, and a ration of other food. Community outreach workers also went into the patient's home.

Rates of weight gain and recovery seemed low, perhaps because mothers were sharing the ready-to-use therapeutic food with siblings at home. Some of the sickest children, with marasmic kwashiorkor, died, perhaps because the diet was faulty for their needs or the treatment at home not precise enough. At the same time, many more children were helped and most remained disease-free during recovery. Mothers were happier, and the percentage of people abandoning treatment was low. Ideally, in Ethiopia, the most vulnerable patients would have also gotten help at small therapeutic feeding centers. But this was not possible. This was not a model for the 10–15 percent of patients who needed intensive medical care. This was a successful model for everyone else. This was a practical, not a perfect solution.

At the Concern Worldwide office in Dublin, Steve energetically draws circles on a piece of paper, showing me how the new concept of Community Therapeutic Care, or CTC, reaches more people and does more good. Each circle represents a local health clinic or food distribution point, with enough circles at the right distance from each other so that people can reach a site easily by walking. This means that a mother will tend to seek help sooner rather than wait until her child is desperately ill. The staff at the center are local, perhaps more sensitive to her concerns and fears. The mother returns home, with food and information, and becomes a teacher herself. When the emergency is over, the staff are still there, the mothers are still there, the clinic is still there, and the community knows more. Health care systems already in place, from government offices to kinship groups, have been strengthened, not abandoned.

All this is linked to the idea of development: creating social support so that chronic malnutrition is no longer the norm and acute malnutrition no longer cyclical. Steve calls it the Holy Grail, a combination of helping in an emergency and helping to prevent emergencies.

The design of a Community Therapeutic Care program is unique to each situation. But there are common principles. The inpatient care of very sick children and adults is not a priority. Resources first go to supplemental feeding programs, outpatient therapeutic care, and mobilizing the community. Healers and village headmen, as well as government agencies, must be included. Traditional songs, dances, and rituals may be part of the educational effort. "Bad feelings" and misperceptions happen easily, and apologies may be necessary. Humility is necessary. In the clinic, and in the home, protocol has to be flexible. The use of local staff means that workers are often illiterate. A color-coded tape that measures the circumference of a child's upper arm will work fine, while a weight-for-height table is too complex. The World Health Organization manual for dealing with children with severe malnutrition or an infection is almost 150 pages long. The protocol for CTC is about three pages.

Community Therapeutic Care seems to focus on children, and I ask Steve what happened to that astonishingly neglected population of adults? "I know," he says." I'm doing the same thing I was complaining about. But when you make a big change like this, it's easier not to change everything all at once. The aid community was used to focusing on children. I made a practical decision."

In partnership with Concern Worldwide, Steve is adapting Community Therapeutic Care to long-term problems of malnutrition and HIV/AIDS—programs that *will* include adults. In the African country of Malawi, 40 percent of the malnourished are also HIV positive, and Community Therapeutic Care will become an entry into the management of that disease. The course of AIDS is clearly aggravated by poor nutrition. Malnourished victims are weaker and die sooner, which creates more hunger in the next generation of children, orphaned before they learn to farm or care for themselves. Good nutrition, on the other hand, with high levels of micronutrients, slows the progress of HIV/AIDS.

Steve abandons his circles and draws a square, with four squares inside. Diarrhea is a common debilitating effect of malnutrition and AIDS, and Valid International, working with Oxford University, has just developed a ready-to-use therapeutic food that has an anti-diarrheal component (including a bacteria from the lactobacillus family, much like what is found in yogurt). They are testing this food in Ethiopia and Malawi. The trial has four groups, hence the four squares: the regular RUTF, also called Plumpynut; Plumpynut with the anti-diarrheal; a second new RUTF made of local agricultural products from Malawi; and the new locally made RUTF with the anti-diarrheal.

In the world of hunger, you have to celebrate success. You have to grab and hold on to any form of success you can find. Malawi is in bad shape. In 2002, food shortages killed over a hundred thousand people in this extremely poor and mostly rural country, a people so vulnerable and malnourished that a single crop failure or season of drought can drive them over the edge. Malawi is one of the worst African countries affected by AIDS, and life expectancy here is expected to drop from a terrible 57.4 to a worse 44.1 years. So when you imagine for these hungry people a ready-to-use therapeutic food—a paste in a sturdy packet that children naturally love because it is made of peanut butter and sugar and oil—when you imagine that this delicious RUTF, packed with micronutrients, also has the ability to control diarrhea, and when you imagine that it can be made regionally, not only more cheaply but also providing income to Malawi farmers, then you have to get excited.

The pilot programs that Concern and Valid International started in Malawi and Ethiopia have been so successful that these governments are moving to adopt Community Therapeutic Care as the national approach, not just for emergencies but as a way to deal with long-term chronic malnutrition.

When I see Steve in Ireland, he has just come back from Bangladesh. His newest idea is to introduce into the urban slums there a version of RUTF that can be sold as snack food. "Snack food?" I repeat a little stupidly. Bangladesh suffers from chronic malnutrition but unlike other countries—Malawi, say, or Ethiopia—people in the cities have a cash economy. "There's always a little change jingling in their pockets," Steve says. He estimates that parents spend about 18 cents a day feeding a child. In Bangladesh, RUTF could be made of local products and sold by local merchants, much like a bag of chips or salted nuts. It would not only generate jobs and income, but Steve estimates that a daily packet of RUTF could easily and affordably add five hundred calories of good nutrition to a child's diet, significantly improving health and growth. Parents would see the difference. They'd rush to buy more. Snack food.

I have a vision. "You'll need to do some marketing. You can get film stars, from India and Bangladesh, on billboards everywhere, eating their tube of paste, a big smile on their faces."

"Good idea," Steve nods to be nice. For a moment we sit quietly in our chairs in the Dublin office of Concern Worldwide. For a moment, we are happy contemplating a future filled with locally made, high-energy, high-caloric, anti-diarrheal, vitamin- and mineral-fortified, ready-to-eat therapeutic food.

AN END
TO HUNGER

IN GUATEMALA, ALMOST HALF OF CHILDREN UNDER the age of five are chronically malnourished. Almost 16 percent suffer from acute malnutrition. Most rural schools only go to third grade, and only a quarter of schoolchildren go on to high school. The poverty and hunger of Guatemala are a result of social choices: civil war, racism, and political oppression. In 1954, the American CIA helped overthrow Guatemala's elected president who had promised to redistribute land to the poor, particularly to the Mayan people, over half the population. Military leaders ruled for the next forty years, and when Marxist-inspired guerrillas resisted, over 150,000 died in a civil war in a country the size of Ohio. The worst massacres occurred in the 1980s when the Guatemalan army, still supported by the American government, destroyed hundreds of villages. Murder and torture were ordinary. Death squads were ordinary. In 1996, the government and remaining guerrillas signed a Peace Accord that promised land reform, public education, a reduction in the army,

and a place in politics for the Mayan majority. Some of these reforms have been achieved, and some have not.

In 1997, I went to Guatemala and spent time with an American
woman who had come to this country as a Peace Corps worker.
Eventually she married a Guatemalan and settled in the village of
Tejar. All across the world, people like this woman find themselves
in poor villages where some version of God speaks to them, "Find
a need and fill it." This woman focused on education. In order to
attend school, Guatemalans must pay for a uniform and supplies,
along with a registration fee. The cost per child per year is about
seventy-five dollars, an impossible sum for most families. My
American went back to her American friends and began a scholarship program that now sends almost a hundred children in Tejar to
school. She found the funds for a one-room public library. She
worked to set up a day care where the young children of working
parents could get meals and medicine. She transformed lives.

While in Guatemala, I also went to a few tourist sites, bird-
watching the Resplendent Quetzal in the cloud forest, hiking
through archaeological ruins in Tikal, where I easily spent seventy-
five dollars many times over. That was my epiphany. I will give
money to the woman in Tejar and to organizations like Concern
Worldwide. I will help—but only so much, only so far. It is not
that I believe these children are less than my own. It is not that I
believe I do not have a responsibility for them. It is just that in a
world of haves and have-nots, I do not want to give up too much
of what I have. I do not want to diminish the complexity and diversity of my life. Instead, I will choose to spend another seventy-
five dollars on myself rather than send another child to school,
and I will choose to do this over and over again. I no longer think
of myself as a good person. I have adjusted to that.

About 800 million chronically malnourished people live in the world. Almost that many experience food shortages and are vulnerable to sudden hunger, the famine caused by drought or war. The truth is that whatever I am willing to do is not enough. Whatever the woman in Tejar is willing to do is not enough. Whatever Steve Collins is willing to do is not enough. It is time for Plan B.

. . .

On the day of the dinner party, when I met with Steve Collins, I also talked to Tom Arnold, the executive director of Concern Worldwide. Tom is a member of the United Nations Hunger Task Force, and he is prepared to make big changes in the world. In 2000, the United Nations adopted eight Millennium Development Goals: (1) Eradicate extreme poverty and hunger; (2) Achieve universal primary education; (3) Promote gender equality and empower women; (4) Reduce child mortality; (5) Improve maternal health; (6) Combat HIV/AIDS, malaria, and other diseases; (7) Ensure environmental sustainability; and (8) Develop a global partnership for development.

These goals are intertwined. They have been broken down into separate targets, eighteen all together. Tom wrestles with Target Two of Goal One: halve between 1990 and 2015 the proportion of people who suffer from hunger.

First, we talk about Concern Worldwide, which began when a group of Irish religious leaders responded to the 1968 famine in Biafra. The Irish have long been active in humanitarian relief, largely because of their missionary work in poor countries and partly because of their history of famine and the Great Hunger of

1845–50. Concern Worldwide grew into an organization that now works in over twenty-six countries, with a 2003 budget of 119 million dollars and a staff of about 4,000 regional workers and 200 Westerners. They focus on people living in absolute poverty. They respond to emergencies and stay for development. Everywhere, they work to improve health. Everywhere, they work to improve education. Everywhere, they work to improve human rights. About 45 percent of their investment goes into livelihood security—agriculture, small loans, community projects—anything that helps people provide for themselves. In Uganda, they build latrines and public water taps. In South Sudan, they distribute seeds, tools, and goats. In Bangladesh, they improve health care for sex workers. In Timor Leste, they encourage small chicken farms.

The job of the U.N. Hunger Task Force has been to look at organizations like Concern Worldwide, at everything that has worked to end hunger and everything that has failed, and to come up with some goals and plans. These plans have to be specific. They have to be measurable. They have to include reports, timetables, and press conferences. The idea is to force accountability. The world can no longer say we do not know what to do—only that we are not doing it.

These are the facts as we know them.

Most of the people who live with hunger are in East and South Asia, 505 million, with the majority in India and China. North Africa and the Near East have 41 million chronically malnourished, Latin America and the Caribbean another 53 million. Sub-Saharan Africa has about 198 million, with the greatest percentage of hungry people in relation to population.

About 50 percent of hungry people are small farmers, 22 percent are the rural landless, 20 percent live in the city, and 8 percent are herders, fishers, or hunters and gatherers. Over a quarter of the hungry have so little food they are unable to work or care for themselves. Cutting across all groups are vulnerable populations: pregnant and nursing women, infants and preschool children, people with HIV/AIDS, and victims of natural disasters or war.

In addition, billions of people have what is called "hidden hunger," a deficiency of micronutrients. Perhaps two billion people are anemic for lack of iron in their diet. Over 100 million children do not get enough Vitamin A and are at risk for blindness.

In Asia, the numbers of hungry people are falling and will continue to fall, probably due to economic growth, political stability, and the Green Revolution. That revolution, over thirty years old, was based on high-yielding varieties of wheat and rice, combined with the use of fertilizers to enrich soil. For some Asian countries, the revolution included irrigation projects, mechanization, changes in crop management, investments in education and research, developments of infrastructure and markets, and growth in the economy. Tom Arnold says that this adds up to "a virtuous circle," a synergy of good things. Since 1960, East Asia has increased its food production per capita by 43 percent and South Asia by 30 percent, while population growth rates have declined. (These statistics say nothing about the distribution of wealth, and a major criticism of the Green Revolution is that it failed to empower the truly poor. As wealthier farmers and businessmen took advantage of the new techniques, poorer farmers were left behind, and the gap between rich and poor widened.)

Sub-Saharan Africa is a different story. Here, food production per capita did not rise. It declined by over 11 percent, while population rose slightly. Both the number and percentage of hungry pcople will continue to increase if trends are not reversed. This is a vicious cycle, Tom Arnold says, fueled by extreme poverty, poor soil, uncertain rainfall, bad roads, inadequate market structure, political oppression, and neglect of the agricultural sector. Conflict and civil war have been major obstacles to development. The widespread horror of AIDS has disrupted families and communities.

If things don't change in Africa and if they don't get better faster elsewhere, the U.N. Millennium Goal will only reach half its goal by 2015. The goal itself is only halfway and leaves 400 million people still hungry.

The Task Force recommends three approaches.

First, mobilize political action to end hunger—globally, nationally, locally, in rich countries and in poor countries.

Second, put in place policies that reduce hunger. Specifically, developing countries must make agricultural and rural investment a priority in their budget; train and support professionals working in the field of agriculture, nutrition, and markets; build and upgrade rural infrastructure; empower women and invest in girls; create safety nets for the vulnerable; provide incentives for the ecologically sound use of natural resources; strengthen property rights and land ownership for the poor; and establish stable and fair trade policies.

Third, start or enhance regional grassroots programs. These programs should improve nutrition for at-risk groups, increase agricultural productivity in small farms, and energize market systems for the poor.

The Task Force is excited about "entry points," the first steps that start the process of transformation. They include efforts to end hunger in early childhood, like Community Therapeutic

Care and school feeding programs. They highlight the education
of women. One study, which looked at sixty-three countries from
1970–96, found that bettering women's education was the single
most important factor in reducing child malnutrition. These first
steps generate synergy. They open the way. Walk out the door
right now and start doing these things. Then follow them up with
"second-order interventions" like agricultural trade reform, less
important in the short term, more important in the long.

None of these parts can operate alone. Political will needs a
practical plan. National policies often bypass the most vulnerable. Local efforts can have a huge impact.

The Task Force urges a "Doubly-Green" revolution for Africa
and mountainous or dry areas of Asia and Latin America. This
revolution would increase production while enhancing the environment. The poorest of the poor would have to be reached, with
the understanding that more food production does not necessarily mean less hunger. The buzzword here is eco-agriculture, and
the terms seem to come from old copies of *Mother Earth News*:
integrated pest management, intercropping, aquaculture, fertil-
izer trees, appropriate technology, sustainability, low-cost. Critics
of the original Green Revolution argue that some of its approaches will have to be reversed, particularly its reliance on
chemical fertilizers, herbicides, and pesticides. Among those critics, there is not much support for genetically engineered crops either, although the debate is not over.

The Task Force has determined a number of hot spots in the
world, places where hunger is persistent and severe. In 2004,
four of these hot spots—Ethiopia, Kenya, Uganda, and Ghana—
stepped forward to be used as test cases for the development of
specific action plans. "These countries are self-selected," Tom

Arnold says. "They are willing to do the work. In Ethiopia, normality is having six million people on food aid. Changing that may mean a radical relooking at policy, at things like the legal system and property rights and the status of women. At the end of the day, it is up to the developing countries themselves. They have to have good governance. They have to want this."

The developed countries have to want this too—enough to double the amount of aid they give, from the current 55 billion to 110 billion dollars a year. They must ensure this aid is used wisely, not for their own political interests, and not for the interests of any elite group. The Task Force suggests that all developed countries contribute 0.7 percent of their gross national product. In 2004, the United States gave 0.15. Ireland gave 0.41. The developed countries can also reform trade practices that hurt farmers in hungry countries, and they can stop dumping cheap agricultural products on these vulnerable markets.

Importantly, powerful countries like the United States have a role in discouraging situations that create hunger. In 1999, the United Nations approved the International Bill of Human Rights, which states that every man, woman, and child has a right to be free from hunger. In this rights-based approach, developed countries would protest hunger just as they do slavery or genocide. This often means promoting democracy. Economist and Nobel prize–winner Amartya Sen has concluded that famine does not happen in places where governments can be held accountable by their people. Frances Moore Lappé, co-author of *World Hunger: Twelve Myths,* agrees: "The root cause of hunger isn't a scarcity of food or land; it's a scarcity of democracy"—within the family, at the village level, at the national level, and in the international arena of commerce and finance.

Tom Arnold believes "the time is ripe. The world is so rich now. There is so much wealth. We can create positive spirals of development. It's a matter of political will. There is just no excuse left."

. . .

That's the big picture. Most of us live in a smaller one. We can change a few lives by giving to Concern Worldwide, to the American woman in Tejar, to those people who are already taking those first steps, building latrines, setting up day cares, and distributing goats. Most of us would be willing to do more if we had a structure that did not involve our personal spending habits. We need economic and political systems that support the goals of the U.N. Hunger Task Force. We need leaders who insist that ending hunger is a priority as important as other national concerns. If necessary, we need to educate these leaders: this is our moral clarity.

In 2004, the coalition National Anti-Hunger Organizations in America came up with a blueprint to end hunger in this country. The first step is to strengthen existing programs. Reach out to the 40 percent of people who are eligible for food stamp benefits but do not receive them. Base benefits on a realistic measure; currently the average benefit is 93 cents per person per meal. Allow people to save for emergencies or other needs while they are receiving food stamps. Reduce the complexity and stigma of getting food stamps. Give food stamps to all legal immigrants in the United States. Expand food for the elderly programs. Make sure that all eligible children get breakfast and lunch in the schools and during school breaks. Provide the Women, Infants, and Children (WIC) program with more resources. The federal and state governments have much to do, but everyone can help—industry, labor, churches, school boards. The second step is to reduce poverty in America. Raise the minimum wage. Expand employment opportunities. Support programs for the working poor. Protect vulnerable groups such as senior citizens and the disabled. This is not rocket science. "The solution to hunger in America is not a secret," said the NAHO. "We have both the knowledge and the tools."

There is no excuse left. We do not have to give up the complexity and diversity of our lives to end hunger. We can have it all. Call us greedy.

. . .

You would not stop there, of course. You would sell your house. You would quit your job. You would move to Ethiopia. You volunteer at the Concern office in Dublin. First you copy files and get coffee. Then you sit by the bed of a dying child. You go back home and declare a hunger-free zone in your town, in your state. You help get a senator elected. You end hunger in America. You wake up at night still grieving. Every man, woman, and child has the right not to be hungry. We can redefine what it means to be human. We can change the future. Millions of children will see a new dawning, something wonderful. You live in mythic time. Your body is huge, and you use it to feed the world.

THE TOP OF
THE MOUNTAIN

H E WAS THE SON OF CALPORNIUS, A DEACON in the Christian Church on the coast of England. Raiders attacked his father's home, killed the servants, and took him to Ireland—where he worked as a slave, often hungry, naked, and cold. It was the beginning of the fifth century AD, and he was sixteen. As an old man, he would write in his autobiography, "But after I came to Ireland—every day I had to herd sheep, and many times a day I prayed—the love of God and His fear came to me more and more, and my faith was strengthened." Sometimes he said a hundred prayers a day and as many at night, getting up before dawn, working through snow, frost, and rain.

Later he would also say that it was hunger itself that brought him to God and that he "lived in death and unbelief until I was severely chastised and really humiliated, by hunger and nakedness." At the same time, this hunger did not weaken him. He felt strong and "there was no sloth in me."

One night, he heard a voice: "It is well that you fast, soon you will go to your own country." Compelled by God, strengthened by hardship, the slave left his master of six years and walked over two hundred miles until he reached a ship ready to sail. Miraculously, the captain gave him passage. After more trials and more weeks without food, he was home among his own people. They received him with joy and urged him never to leave again.

But he kept having visions. A man named Victoricus appeared in a dream with "countless letters," the voices of the Irish begging him to return with the message of Christ. On other nights, God spoke to him and called him "the apple of my eye." In the meantime, he was made a deacon and then a bishop, and finally he left his family and country for the last time, on his own accord, to return to the people from whom he had once escaped. He went back to teach "the barbarians" the Gospel, and he stayed thirty years until his death, probably around 460 AD. Perhaps a quarter million people lived in Ireland at this time, mostly herders and small farmers with an oral tradition and established laws. These Celts were ruled by warrior-kings advised by druids and a heritage of ritual and magic. One by one, across Ireland, Saint Patrick converted them—poor men and poor women, kings and slaves, sailors and traders. His work laid the foundation for the church to come, so that a hundred years later you could say this was a Christian land.

For four centuries, Christianity had strengthened the link between fasting, hunger, and sanctity. Fasting brought Christians together, prepared the way for the greater feast, healed disease, and cast out demons. Fasting made women pure and men obedient. Saint Jerome had admonished, "Let your companions be those who are thin with fasting, of pallid countenance" and other Christians agreed, "For fasting is the life of the angels, and the one who makes use of it has angelic rank."

Saint Patrick may have brought these ideas to his adopted land, but not as something new. The druids also understood hunger as a spiritual state, with magical properties. Moreover, hunger had a legal dimension and could be used to coerce and chastise. Early Irish law described the practice of *troscad*, fasting against a person of high rank in order to pressure him to pay a debt or right a wrong. Probably the accuser fasted on the accused's doorstep, waiting there morning and night, morning and night—a dour, self-righteous package. The rules of *troscad* were complex. Simply put: if the accused agreed to settle the case, the faster had to eat. If the accused held out against a properly conducted fast, he lost his legal rights in society. Most historians believe that by the fifth century any threatened fast to the death had been ritualized into abstinence from sunrise to sunset. During this period, the accused was obliged to fast as well, unless he was willing to give justice to the claim.

For the Irish, hunger was readily seen as power: magical, moral, and legal. Saint Patrick used it as power, too. One day he climbed a steep hill on the coast of western Ireland, a place where people had lived and worshipped since 300 BC. Patrick's habit was to perform Christian rituals at long-established sacred sites. Now, when he reached the summit, he fasted for forty days. According to legend, at the end of this time—as his ecstasy mounted and the ketones sparked in his brain, as the angels gloried, as the power burst from his fingers and toes—Saint Patrick raised his staff and drove out all the snakes from Ireland. The ground crawled with a flood of reptiles slithering, sliding, soaring over the cliff into the ocean below. The legend does not explain whether snakes were a real plague in the country or a metaphor for human sin. In either case, this was a grand event, and this was where a church would be built, somewhere between the fifth and ninth century, on the mountain called Croagh Patrick.

The pilgrimages started later. Men and women often walked barefoot up Croagh Patrick, stopping to do penance at three stations along the way. Up until the 1970s, thousands of pilgrims did this on certain nights, with shoes and without, each carrying a candle or flashlight so that a ribbon of light ascended upward. Tens of thousands still make this pilgrimage in large groups or alone, and a guidebook to Ireland warns that the mountain will be particularly busy during the summer holiday season. Otherwise, "hope for that scarce commodity, a fine day."

My nineteen-year-old daughter and I walked up before the holiday rush, and we had that rare commodity, too, a fine day. The trail begins from the main road, past a little café, through a leafy lane, along a tumbling stony creek, by low stone walls, by grazing sheep, by fields of heather and stone, onto a stony path unnaturally wide for all those pilgrims. The upper part of the cone-shaped mountain is white quartzite fractured into a mantle of scree, which makes climbing difficult even with shoes. It will be over two hours, with a twenty-five hundred feet rise in elevation, before we reach the top. But we don't know that yet, enamored with the sheep and blue sky. The last half hour is very steep and the footing poor, with minor rock slides. The top, we begin to understand, might not really exist. This might be purgatory or worse. This might be a mountain's idea of a joke. Then we are there, and the view looks north over the green Irish coast and Clew Bay with its turquoise water and legendary 356 islands, one for every day of the year. The deep-blue Atlantic Ocean fills the west, and it is not just as far as you can see, but as far as you would ever want to see.

Walking back, rolling down Croagh Patrick, you might as well roll down Irish history. Saint Patrick established churches and abbeys at holy Celtic sites, centers of scholarship that would make Ireland a light during the coming Dark Ages. Vikings attacked the country in a series of bloody raids, until the hero-chieftain Brian Boru defeated them and was recognized as king of Ireland. In the eleventh century, England also tried to conquer Ireland, beginning an eight-hundred-year struggle between the two countries.

More battles, more invasions, more defeats. In 1497, there were reports of a major famine, with people eating "food unbecoming to mention." From 1529–41, Henry the Eighth broke with Rome, set up the Church of England, and declared himself king of Ireland. In 1598, Sir Edmund Spenser told Queen Elizabeth, "Until Ireland can be famished, it cannot be subdued." The English seized Irish lands like those held by the Kelleys in my family and "planted" them with Scotsmen, like the Russells in my husband's family. In 1649, an Irish rebellion was crushed by Oliver Cromwell. Later in England, Protestants successfully rose up against the Catholic Church.

Now, Catholics in Ireland—the majority of the population—were excluded from voting, holding office, owning property, and practicing their religion. Many became landless tenants living in extreme poverty. When the potato crop failed from 1739–41, a quarter million people died, or one-tenth the population. In 1798, the political economist Thomas Malthus explained famines like this as a check on population growth. Malthus believed that the human species, if unchecked, would reproduce geometrically and disastrously. His observation that plants and animals in nature produce far more offspring than can survive became a key idea in Darwin's theory of evolution.

In 1800, Ireland and England were politically joined, with the Irish given minority seats in the English Parliament. The new free trade between the countries allowed England to dump its surplus goods, and Ireland's nascent industry collapsed. From 1816–42, there were repeated local failures of the potato crop. Catholics received the right to vote but the fee for voting was raised from 40 shillings to 40 pounds. In 1844, more English soldiers were stationed in Ireland than in India. In 1845, the potato fields of Ireland turned black. During the Great Hunger or *An Gorta Mor* of 1845–50, at least a million people died and over two million eventually emigrated. The country and culture of Ireland would be irrevocably changed.

Rolling down Croagh Patrick, the view is gorgeous, blue-green water and green land. You smile and wave at the pilgrims and tourists going up the mountain, reassuring them that they, too, will reach the top. They smile and wave back. You pass by the gurgling stony creek and the lamb bleating for its ma, and the little café where you can get tea and scones, and across the road that runs by the bay, and now you are at a rolling park with grass and a pond and the National Famine Memorial. This great bronze sculpture is a ship, not life-size, but still large, with three masts rising over twenty feet high. From mast to mast, from hull to prow, skeletons stretch and splay out like rigging, the bones of their arms and legs as thin as rope. Simultaneously, they seem to crawl by choice and to be lashed against their will, the eerie ghosts of what came to be called coffin ships. As people left Ireland, they often sailed away in these rickety vessels, where they were jammed together like human ballast. The coffin ships frequently sank or reached their destination with half the passengers dead of dehydration and disease. Even so, they were preferred by those who felt their other choice was to stay on land and starve.

Based on exports from 1600–1845, Ireland's agricultural production had actually boomed in the years before the Great Hunger. Irish farmers were producing more things to sell, such as animal products, wheat, and barley, and more things to eat at home, such as potatoes, pigs, oats, and poultry. The potato helped make this abundance possible. Related to tomatoes and peppers, the potato originated in the high mountains of Peru and Bolivia. Sailors who ate the vegetable on their voyages back from the New World didn't get scurvy, and by the late seventeenth century, the potato was a widespread field crop in Ireland, on its way to becoming a staple. With only a spade and strong pair of arms, a large crop of potatoes could be produced magically from a small piece of land. Potatoes helped break up the soil for sowing and grew in wet, poor areas—like the high bogs and mountains of western Ireland—where nothing else did. Potatoes could be fed to animals, and they were a healthy, good-tasting food for humans too. An adult male worker in Ireland might consume fourteen pounds of potatoes a day, with salt, and some cabbage and fish. Such meals supplemented with buttermilk and oatmeal were a reasonably nutritious diet, better than what many other Europeans were eating.

Cheap food meant a cheap labor force paid a "potato wage" of a plot of land. These marginalized workers had access to free fuel like peat and free housing made of local materials. They married early and had large families. Between 1790 and 1840, the population of Ireland increased from five million to eight and a half. In the countryside, most people still spoke the Irish language, not English, with longstanding traditions of hospitality and boisterous community events.

On the eve of the Great Hunger, over a third of the Irish had come to rely on potatoes as their main food. Some were landless laborers. Others rented from Irish and English landlords, and the rent was high, as much as 100 percent higher than in England. These farmers were often on the verge of eviction, growing cash crops like corn to pay the rent and potatoes to feed the family. In other areas of Ireland, grains could hardly grow at all, and people subsisted completely on potatoes. The few industrialized areas of Ireland were declining or in the process of mechanization. Large parts of Ireland had no cash economy at all. One visitor to Galway noted that "so little do the people know of the commercial value of money that they are constantly in the habit of pawning it." Even before the famine of 1845, an estimated two million Irish periodically went hungry as a matter of course, every season, every year, a huge population of people already wretched, already beggared, already evicted, already widowed, already orphaned, already hungry.

The potato blight first appeared in the United States in 1843, probably brought over with potato stock from Peru. From a single diseased plant, the fungal infestation reproduces through millions of spores carried to another plant by wind or water, attacking the leaves and stalk and then penetrating the soil to spread through the tuber. The spores require a mild, damp environment. They germinate and send out radiating fungus tubes that drain the plant's juices, devouring it from within and choking its systems of getting food and air. The leaves darken and wither. There is fermentation and decay. In a short time, fine-looking potatoes stored or in the ground melt into slimy, foul-smelling blobs of corruption.

In 1845, in Ireland, a third of the potatoes harvested in the fall were diseased. The British government set up a commission to investigate, although an understanding of the blight would not come for many years. The prime minister used the crisis as a way to repeal restrictions on the importation of grain, which infuriated English farmers. Some British officials saw the famine as Providence or God's will. Some saw this Providence as an opportunity to reorder Irish society, ending the people's dependency on the potato and breaking up the numerous small farms into large, modern, "efficient" estates. In this scheme, grain would naturally become the dominant crop, the economy would soar, and the lazy, rebellious Irish would be saved from themselves. Eventually the British became fully committed to a policy of laissez-faire, letting each individual pursue his own economic interest, without government interference.

The English also wanted Irish landowners to be responsible for their poor. The government should provide transitional aid only. To this end, the British purchased a minimal amount of corn to feed the hungry and determined that the food would not be given away but released slowly into the market, at cost, to relief organizations. Some public works programs were set up, badly run, and punitive in nature, and some workhouses readied. Exports of food were not banned since this would only discourage the production of food. The larger goal was not to relieve suffering but to allow the market system to operate freely and thus change Irish society for the better. Landowners would rise to the occasion. Merchants and businessmen would rise to the occasion.

Relatively few Irish starved in the first year of the famine. This was not the case in other parts of Europe that experienced the potato blight. Tens of thousands died in Belgium and the Netherlands. English laborers in 1845 were also at risk, for they were well on their way to becoming dependent on the potato too.

With hope, and without much choice, the Irish replanted and waited for the crop of 1846. It did not come. One priest reported that he had traveled from Cork to Dublin and seen the fields blooming luxuriantly; on his return, however, he "beheld with sorrow one wide waste of putrefying vegetation. In many places the wretched people were seated on the fences of their decaying gardens, wringing their hands and wailing bitterly the destruction that had left them foodless." That fall, three-quarters of the crops were destroyed. The price of food rose astronomically, and in a few areas, food could hardly be found at all. Instead, people ate nettles and weeds, blackberries and roots, seaweed and limpets, dogs and rats. They boiled cabbage leaves. They forced down the diseased and rotting potatoes. They ate carrion. They ate grass. They ate the hard unprocessed corn given out by the British government, which one official noted was about as useful as a ration of river sand.

In 1847, the British admitted that their work programs had been an expensive failure: the projects were ill-advised and hungry people made poor laborers. Now the government tried soup kitchens, another temporary measure. Too little, too late, the free soup still reduced mortality until the kitchens were closed in September, again with the idea that local property owners should be responsible for their poor. For these landlords, every destitute non-paying tenant now represented a tax or cost. Already squeezed, the landlords responded with mass evictions. Houses were "tumbled" and tens of thousands of families sent away to live in banks and ditches, to find their way to overcrowded workhouses or to die on the side of the road. Landlords also evicted tenants with the idea of clearing the land for a more modern form of agriculture.

The potato blight spared the 1847 crops but reappeared in 1848, 1849, and 1850. The government gave less and less aid despite the increasing need. Private charity, which had included generous contributions from Irish already in Canada and the United States, had reached its limit. The British Association for Relief ran out of funds. Even the Quakers abandoned their work in 1849, saying that only the state could deal with the enormity of the disaster. Those Irish who could often chose to emigrate. Some had their fares paid by landlords, a more beneficent form of eviction.

The Great Hunger was not a secret. Journalists, travelers, and missionaries described horrific scenes: houses filled with the dying, mothers half-naked, babies screaming in pain, crowds of wolfish gaunt men, corpses piled on the street. These accounts included all the physical signs of starvation, the wizened and shrunken children with marasmus—their bones deformed, their "skin black like an oven," their faces covered with a fine hair so that they looked like "monkeys"—and the victims with kwashiorkor, then called dropsy, "swollen and ripening for the grave."

Disease followed hunger. Scurvy was a new plague for people accustomed to a diet high in Vitamin C. Their joints swelled. Their gums became spongy. Occasionally they died of bleeding into the heart muscle or brain. The blindness caused by Vitamin A deficiency was common in the workhouses. A lack of niacin and Vitamin B was also something new, its early symptoms easily confused with typhus. More people, of course, died of typhus first. Carried by lice, the typhus bacterium enters the blood-stream and damages blood vessels, especially in the skin and brain: the victim starts with a rash, turns dark blue, suffers ago-nizing sores, stinks terribly, and becomes delirious. Other infec-tions included relapsing fever, bacillary dysentery, measles, scarlet fever, tuberculosis, smallpox, and influenza. Cholera be-came epidemic in 1849. According to one chronicler of the time, over half a million people died of disease from 1844–51. The real number is probably higher.

Throughout the famine, ships of corn and barley left Ireland to be sold elsewhere. Although imports of food, donated or bought by relief organizations, exceeded exports, the fact that the government would not ban exports aroused a deep and abiding anger. Convoys of grain on their way to harbor had to be guarded by military de-tachments. Then, as now, hunger was a matter of entitlement. Food was available, but the poor were not entitled to that food. They did not grow it. They did not have a legal claim to it as a pension or form of social welfare. They did not have the money to buy it.

The Great Hunger was not inevitable. On one hand, the potato blight was a natural disaster, and the food shortage was real. Even if exports had been prohibited, even if all that food had been dis-tributed to the needy, it would not have been enough. Still, many more people would have survived if the British government and Irish elite had intervened effectively. In the end, from 1845–50, the British Treasury spent slightly over seven million pounds for relief, contrasted to the twenty million pounds they had earlier given West Indian slave owners as compensation for emancipat-ing their slaves or the seventy million pounds they would soon spend on the Crimean War of 1854–56. The famine could be called a failure of capitalism. Economic ideology had prevailed, as well as the usual suspects of greed, apathy, ignorance, and fear. (For Ireland was an enemy always too close, always ready to harbor England's foes and rebel against her rule. "With the money they get from our relief funds," one officer fretted, "they buy arms.") Some people did respond with great compassion, and these included British officials and Irish landlords. Doctors and clergy also died at a tremendous rate, not from starvation, but from their attempts to help the sick.

After the famine of 1845–50, much of the native Irish culture—its language and folk customs—declined. Unlike other famines, however, unlike most, this one would not be forgotten. The emigrants who left Ireland took with them their memories, their rage, and their loyalties. Manhattan, New York, has a five-million dollar monument that includes a reconstructed nineteenth-century Irish cottage, brought to America rock by rock, nestled in sixty-two varieties of native Irish grasses. Boston has a million-dollar memorial park, with emaciated bronze figures. Cambridge has another. So do Philadelphia and Quebec. There are at least seven monuments in Ireland, and a variety of parks, plaques, sculptures, commemorations, and remembrances.

In a collection of stories about the famine, actor Gabriel Byrne remembered the stories his mother told him, that she got from her mother, told by her mother in turn. The images of starvation and death haunted his childhood. Once his father pointed to an empty road, asking him what he saw. "Nothing, I replied. Look close, he urged, and you will see not just the trees and the hedgerows but the ghosts of all the people who have ever walked this road. Every street, every road is crowded with them. The past is always with us, the earth absorbs our blood and our tears."

In a novel by Irish writer Nuala O'Faolin, a character says briskly, "If you and I are sitting here in a warm room having a nice talk, we have to ask ourselves how our own people survived. What did our people do at the time, that you and I came to be born? Anyone who had a field of cabbages or turnips put a guard on it to keep off the starving. We were those guards."

In 1992, the President of Ireland, Mary Robinson, visited Baidoa, Somalia. She sat beside a woman too weak to lift the small bundle of her child, a sick baby with sores and flies crawling over his mouth and eyes. At a press conference, Robinson spoke emotionally, "I have an inner sense of justice. It has been deeply offended. . . . I felt shamed by what I saw, shamed, shamed. . . . What are we doing that we have not got a greater conscience?"

The legacy of the Great Hunger is multiple: anger, guilt, an inner sense of justice. Yet the story of the famine is perhaps most surprising, and most surprisingly hopeful, in the context of Ireland today. Over a hundred and fifty years later, you will leave Croagh Patrick and the National Famine Memorial and drive back to the small tourist town of Westport, where you will pay a fair amount for the cheapest bed and breakfast, and where the breakfast will be enormous, much more than you can eat. Over a hundred and fifty years later, Ireland has one of the highest standards of living in Europe, and thus in the world. Its economy is called the Celtic Tiger. Its people are rich in material goods, in food, in heritage, in scenery. Like many visitors, you don't ever want to leave.

Something happened here, a virtuous circle. If you are talking to people about hunger, hunger in Somalia and in the past, if you are walking the famine roads and visiting the famine museums, there is a subtle resonance, an optimism you dare not make too explicit. Things got better.

. . .

In Northern Ireland, I go from mural to mural. In Derry, the giant images of barbwire and children wearing gas masks overlook the site of Bloody Sunday, where in 1972 British policemen killed fourteen peaceful protesters. In Belfast, the murals line certain streets and signal the separation between Protestant and Catholic neighborhoods. My taxicab driver tells me that the city is painting over the goriest pictures, the guns and dripping blood that children walking home from school should not have to look at every day. He points to a hospital, remarking how its specialty became the repair of bones damaged by bullets, what with so many soldiers shooting civilians and civilians shooting policemen and all the knee-capping that went on. Of course, he remembers the hunger strikes very well, the ten men who died over twenty years ago in the prison not far from here. We go to a memorial of black marble honoring their sacrifice. The flowers in the vases along the wall are fresh.

South of Belfast, still in Northern Ireland, Armagh is a beautiful town with two beautiful cathedrals, both named for Saint Patrick. In one of its neighborhoods, in a row of small brick homes, I find a mural of Bobby Sands and Francis Hughes and Raymond McCreesh and Patsy O'Hara and all the rest. Their floating heads surround a poem and central figure, possibly Brian Boru with his long reddish hair and silver sword, the victorious warrior-king. The ten men died fasting on the British doorstep, the ancient *troscad*. Hunger was part of their mythology, their mythic past, their mythic future. Francis Hughes wrote of his "unshakable belief that we are a noble race and that chains and bonds have no part in us." Francis Hughes was a martyr and a terrorist. Although his politics repulse me, I find myself admiring his hunger.

Hunger cannot be ignored. Hunger signals you to take what you need. Hunger makes you reach out your hand. Your brain, your stomach, your cells hunger. They break down matter and transform it into something else, the gestalt of your life. You cannot live without hunger. You cannot live with hunger. Hunger begins your exchange with the world.

One day, according to legend, Saint Patrick wanted something from God, a favor for himself or his people. For reasons unknown, God was reluctant to grant the saint's request. So Patrick went on a hunger strike, a *troscad* unto death. Repeatedly, angelic messengers begged him to break his fast. They implored. They sang. They remonstrated. But Patrick was steadfast. Patrick would not eat. Against this hunger, even God gave in.

SELECTED REFERENCES
AND NOTES

CHAPTER ONE: THE HUNGER ARTISTS

The idea that the mechanisms of food addiction and drug addiction have some physical similarities can be found in a number of articles, including Roy Wise, "Drug Self-Administration Viewed as Ingestive Behavior," *Appetite* 28 (1997), pages 1–5. The article nicely begins, "The brain circuitry and chemical message systems that mediate addiction evolved long before the phenomenon of addiction itself. Addiction is a recent evolutionary development; it emerged with the human mastery of fire, the hypodermic syringe, and the bottle and cork. The receptors for addictive drugs and neural circuitry in which these receptors are imbedded, on the other hand, emerged with animal life itself and have, from their inception, been associated with ingestive behavior." This theme is continued in Clifford B. Saper, et al, "The Need to Feed: Homeostatic and Hedonic Control of Eating," *Neuron* 36 (October 10, 2002), pages 199–211. The authors mention that "opioid receptors play key roles in both feeding and reward" and that "mice that genetically lack the ability to produce dopamine normally die of starvation." Serotonin also has well-recognized influences on feeding and mood. The statement that "dopaminergic brain circuitry originally developed to subserve eating behavior" is in Angelo Del Parigi, et al, "Are We Addicted to Food?" *Obesity Research* 11, no. 4 (April 2003), pages 493–95.

A good book to read on hunger and history is Lucille Newman and William Cosgrove, *Hunger in History: Food Shortage, Poverty, and Deprivation* (Cambridge: Blackwell Publishers, 1990).

How long any one human can survive without food is variable. One estimate for a well-fed young man is eighty days, stated in Christopher Saudek and Philip Felig, "The Metabolic Events of Starvation," *The American Journal of Medicine* 60 (January 1976), pages 117–26. Nine out of the ten Irish hunger strikers died between fifty-seven and seventy-three days, however, after losing 40 percent of their body weight, as noted by M. Elia in "Hunger Disease," *Clinical Nutrition* 19, no. 6 (2000). My statement of sixty days is another estimated average time, based on my readings.

The quotes from "A Hunger Artist" come from Franz Kafka, *The Complete Stories* (New York: Schoken Books, 1946).

Information about Succi can be found in many places, including the excellent book by Walter Vandereycken and Ron van Deth, *From Fasting Saints to Anorexic Girls, the History of Self-starvation* (New York: New York University Press, 1996). This book is also the source for the quote and the material on the hunger artist in Germany who sat under a glass bell, "a kind of human skeleton in dress-jacket, smoking cigarettes, with a glass of water in front of him on a little marble table."

Material about David Blaine's fast can be found at his extensive website chronicling the event. Other accounts are in such news magazine and newspaper articles as "Empty Box," *The Economist* (September 27, 2003) and "Blaine sips magic potion," *The New York Daily News* (October 21, 2003).

The story of the longest fast is in W. K. Stewart and Laura W. Fleming, "Features of a successful therapeutic fast of 382 days' duration," *Postgraduate Medical Journal* 49 (March 1973), pages 203–09.

The quotes by Knut Hamsun come from *Hunger*, translated and with an afterword by Robert Bly (New York: Farrar, Straus, and Giroux, 1967). The quote by Robert Bly is in the afterword. The quotes by George Orwell come from *Down and Out in Paris and London* (New York: Harcourt and Brace, 1933).

There is a wealth of information on calorie restriction. A place to start is the website of the Calorie Restriction Society, http://www.caloriere-striction.org. For some good outside overviews, look at Jerry Adler and Anne Underwood, "Starve Your Way to Health," *Newsweek* (January 19, 2004), pages 51–54; David Schardt, "Eat Less and Live Longer?" *Nutrition Action* 30, no. 7 (September 2003), pages 1–7; Leonie K. Heilbronn and Eric Ravussin, "Calorie Restriction and aging: review of the literature and implications for studies in humans," *American Journal of Clinical Nutrition* 78 (2003), pages 361–69; Laura Johannes, "Lean Times," *The Wall Street Journal Online* (June 3, 2002); and Edward Masoro, "Caloric restriction and aging: an update," *Experimental Gerontology* 35 (2000), pages 299–305. I also communicated personally with Eric Ravussin.

The study concerning fasting mice has been widely reported. Look at R. Michael Anson, et al, "Intermittent fasting dissociates beneficial effects of dietary restriction on glucose metabolism and neuronal resistance to injury from calorie intake," *Proceedings of the National Academy of Sciences in the United States of America* 100, no. 10 (May 13, 2003), pages 6216–20.

Some of the statistics on famine were taken from "Hunger Disease." The quote from Egypt was also quoted in this article, the original source is J. Cornell, *The Great International Disaster Book* (New York: Scribners, 1976).

CHAPTER TWO: EIGHTEEN HOURS

For a general overview of digestion, I recommend Sherwin B. Nuland, *The Wisdom of the Body* (New York: Alfred A. Knopf, 1997). I also used Arthur C. Guyton and John E. Hall, *Textbook of Medical Physiology*, 10th ed. (Philadelphia: W. B. Saunders Company, 2000).

The study on two severely amnesiac patients is in Paul Rozin, et al, "What Causes Humans to Begin and End a Meal?" *Psychological Science* 9, no. 5 (September 1998), pages 392–96.

A few words about insulin and its multiple roles: insulin facilitates the passage of glucose into the cells. When people do not produce insulin or when they become resistant to its effect, their blood sugar level shoots up and remains high, since the glucose is not being made available. Your body is starving for glucose even though, ironically, you have lots of glucose in your blood system. That, in itself, is a problem. Too much glucose in the blood can dehydrate cells and damage blood vessels. Insulin also stimulates the liver to form glycogen out of excess glucose, a way of storing energy for later use. Glucagon is the hormone that tells the liver to convert its supply of glycogen back into glucose. The names are annoyingly confusing since they are so similar. Insulin regulates fat metabolism, too, inhibiting the release of fatty acids from fat tissue and prompting the body to store fat rather than burn it. The reverse happens—your body releases fatty acids and you burn fat, not glucose—when insulin levels are low. (The membrane of a resting muscle cell does not easily allow glucose to pass through unless stimulated by insulin, as in right after a meal. In heavy or moderate exercise, muscle cells also use glucose instead of fatty acids.)

The quotes from Michael Gershon come from *The Second Brain* (New York: HarperPerennial, 1999). This is a fun book with lots of interesting information.

Some of the latest material on ghrelin can be found in Masamitsu Nakazato, et al, "A role for ghrelin in the central regulation of feeding," *Nature* 408, no. 11 (January 2001), pages 194–97; John Travis, "The Hunger Hormone?" *Science News* 161 (February 16, 2002), pages 107–8; Michael D. Lemonick, "Lean and Hungrier," *Time* (June 3, 2002), page 54; and Julie Eisenstein, "Ghrelin, Update 2003," *Nutrition Reviews* 61, no. 3 (March 2003). The study on ghrelin and the buffet table is in A. M. Wren, "Ghrelin Enhances Appetite and Increases Food Intake in Humans," *The Journal of Clinical Endocrinology and Metabolism* 86, no. 12 (2001), pages 5992–95.

The term recessive body is used in Drew Leder, *The Absent Body* (Chicago: University of Chicago Press, 1990). The material from Lewis Thomas is quoted in this book, page 49, as is the phrase from Aristotle, the "ensouled" body, page 47. The quote about the "repeatedly reconstructed biological state" comes from Antonio R. Damasio, *Descartes'*

Error: Emotion, Reason, and the Human Brain (New York: G. P. Putnam's Sons, 1994), page 227.

My exploration of appetite and satiety included Deborah Lupton, *Food, the Body, and the Self* (London: Sage Publications, 1996) and S. T. Kristensen, "Social and cultural perspectives on hunger, appetite, and satiety," *European Journal of Clinical Nutrition* 54 (2000), pages 473–78.

A discussion of neophobia—including mention of the aversion of a Jewish group to breaking dietary laws—can be found in Patricia Pliner and Marcia L. Pelchat, "Neophobia in Humans and the Special Status of Goods of Animal Origin," *Appetite* 16 (1991), pages 205–18. The study that used video games is Patricia Pliner and Nancy Melo, "Food Neophobia in Humans: Effects of Manipulated Arousal and Individual Differences in Sensation Seeking," *Physiology and Behavior* 61, no. 2 (1997), pages 331–35.

Although hungry people don't commonly resort to cannibalism, one famous and recent exception took place in 1972, when a plane of Uruguayan rugby players, relatives, and friends crashed in the Andes Mountains. The survivors lived for months by eating the frozen bodies of the dead. In this case, the tough-minded young men were able to break the old rules and create a new, temporary culture. One athlete compared the act of eating the dead bodies to Communion.

The final quote is from *The Absent Body*, page 42.

CHAPTER THREE: THIRTY-SIX HOURS

Information on Angelo Del Parigi's work came from interviews and personal correspondence, as well as Jean-François Gautier, et al, "Effect of Satiation on Brain Activity in Lean and Obese Women," *Obesity Research* 9, no. 11 (November 2001), pages 676–84; Angelo Del Parigi, et al, "Neuroimaging and Obesity," *Annual New York Academy of Sciences* 967 (2002), pages 389–97; and Angelo Del Parigi, et al, "Sex differences in the human brain's response to hunger and satiation," *American Journal of Clinical Nutrition* 75 (2002), pages 1017–22.

The estimates of our stored calories or savings bank comes from "The Metabolic Events of Starvation."

Information on the first trials concerning leptin is in many sources, including the well-researched Ellen Ruppel Shell, *The Hungry Gene: The Science of Fat and the Future of Thin* (New York: Atlantic Monthly Press, 2002), as well as articles like Marion E. Glick, "Leptin Helps Body Regulate Fat, Links to Diet," Rockefeller Education Public Information Release (October 31, 1995) and "Friedman Receives Bristol-Myers Squibb Award," Rockefeller Education Public Information Release, *News and Notes* 12, no. 23 (June 8, 2001). I took my list of countries with half the adult population overweight or obese from Shell's excellent book.

The study on cancer cachexia mouse models being given ghrelin is from T. Hanada, et al, "Anti-cachectic effect on ghrelin in nude mice bearing human melanoma cells," *Biochemical and Biophysical Research Communications* 301, no. 2, (February 2003), pages 275–79.

The story about the children missing leptin was told in *The Hungry Gene*.

Information about Prader-Willi can be found at the website for the Prader-Willi Syndrome Association or http://www.pwsausa.org. I also recommend Kathleen Megowan, "Are You Hungry?" *Discover* (September 2002), page 23; and "Hunger hormone gone awry?" *Science News* (July 6, 2002), page 162.

Statistics on the hungry in America can be found in many sources, including organizations like America's Second Harvest at www.hunger-day.org or Food Resources Action Committee at http://www.frac.org. Statistics from government agencies such as the U.S.D.A. or from hunger advocacy groups all tell the same story.

The information on the Roadrunner Food Bank comes from personal interviews and correspondence. If you are interested in more information or in making a contribution, write to Roadrunner Food Bank of New Mexico, 2645 Baylor Drive, S.E., Albuquerque, New Mexico 87106 or call 505–247–2052, ext 101.

CHAPTER FOUR: SEVEN DAYS

More information on ketones and ketosis can be found in Richard L. Veech, et al, "Ketone Bodies, Potential Therapeutic Uses," *Life* 51

(2001), pages 241–47 and in Ben Harder, "Ketones to the Rescue," *Science News* 164 (December 13, 2003), pages 376–77. The use of ketosis in epilepsy is specifically discussed in Stephen L. Kinsman, et al, "Efficacy of the Ketogenic Diet for Intractable Seizure Disorders: review of 58 cases," *Epilepsia* 33, no. 6 (1992), pages 1132–36; John Freeman, et al, "The efficacy of the ketogenic diet—1998: A prospective evaluation of intervention in 150 children," *Pediatrics* 102, no. 6 (December 1998), pages 1358–63; and Eileen P. G. Vining, et al, "Seizures Decrease Rapidly After Fasting," *Arch Pediatrics of Adolescent Medicine* 153 (September 1999), pages 946–49.

In the popular Atkins diet—eating lots of protein as well as fat, with very few carbohydrates—fatty acids also become a substitute for glucose. Here, ketosis is seen as fat-burning and desirable, a kind of paradise where you can eat lobster, butter, bacon, and cream and still lose weight. However, no one has studied the long-term effect of ketosis on the brain or kidneys, which in the Atkins diet work overtime to deal with acids caused by fat breakdown and protein metabolism. In personal correspondence, Dr. Richard Veech warned against ketosis in people with pre-existing heart conditions since the elevation of free fatty acids in the blood affects "the transcription of uncoupling proteins," which can induce cardiac abnormalities like unstable angina and cardiac arrhythmia.

For one description of what happens in complete water fasting, read Joel Fuhrman, M.D., *Fasting and Eating for Health* (New York: St. Martin's Griffin, 1995). I also looked at articles like Daryl DeVivo, et al, "Chronic Ketosis and Cerebral Metabolism," *Annuals of Neurology* 3, no. 4 (April 1978), pages 329–37; S. G. Hasselbalch, "The Human Brain Utilizes Ketone Bodies After Three Days of Starvation," *Journal of Cerebral Blood Flow and Metabolism* 13 (1993), page 579; Steen G. Hasselbalch, et al, "Brain Metabolism During Short-Term Starvation in Humans," *Journal of Cerebral Blood Flow and Metabolism* 14 (1994), pages 125–31; and Ronaldo Ferraris, et al, "Intestinal transport during fasting and malnutrition," *Annual Review of Nutrition* 20 (2000), pages 195–219.

The story of the Buddha is from many sources. I like Karen Armstrong, *Buddha* (New York: Penguin Putnam, 2001). More information on how Tamils use fasting is in Elizabeth Fuller Collins, *Pierced by Muragan's Lance* (De Kalb, Illinois: Northern Illinois University Press, 1997), page 56.

I quote the Taoist story from Burton Watson, *Chuang Tzu, Basic Writing* (New York: Columbia University Press, 1964), page 127.

Fasting in various religions comes from a variety of general sources. The quote from Long Standing Bear Chief is from *Ni-Kso-Ko-Wa: Blackfoot Spirituality, Traditions, Values, and Beliefs* (Browning, Montana: Spirit Talk Press, 1992), page 41.

The quote from the writer we call pseudo-Athanasius is in a number of sources, including Caroline Walker Bynum, *Holy Feast and Holy Fast, the Religious Significance of Food to Medieval Women* (Berkeley: University of California Press, 1987), page 36. This is a wonderful book about medieval life, female saints, and the symbolic language of food and fasting. It also contains some information about modern female saints such as Theresa Neumann.

Material about Saint Jerome and the quote from him concerning the twelve-year-old Asella come from another great book—Teresa M. Shaw, *The Burden of the Flesh: Fasting and Sexuality in Early Christianity* (Minneapolis: Fortress Press, 1998), page 106. The philosopher John Cassian who wrote of the "quality of our purity" is also discussed in Shaw's book, pages 112–24, as are various Christian vices such as gluttony. The other quotes by Jerome can be found in Charles Christopher Mierow, *The Letters of Jerome* (New York: Newman Press, 1963), pages 148 and 158.

Ideas about fasting and early Christianity are much more complex and rich than I can present in a short space. For example, in *The Burden of the Flesh*, Shaw believes that medieval Christians saw the ascetic body as a sign of "both the original, pure human body of paradise and the incorruptible condition of the paradise to come. Ascetic discipline looks back to the garden and forward to the kingdom. By fasting, as by chastity and renunciation of 'the world,' the ascetic aligns herself or himself with ideal humanity—the perfect, trouble-free humanity created 'in the image of God' and the future humanity restored to that image."

A number of books discuss the female saints, including Rudolph Bell, *Holy Anorexia* (Chicago: University of Chicago Press, 1985); *Holy Feast and Holy Fast, the Religious Significance of Food to Medieval Women*; and *The Burden of the Flesh*. The quotes by Catherine of Siena were in *Holy Anorexia*.

The material concerning fasting maids came from many sources, notably the seminal Joan Jacobs Brumberg, *Fasting Girls: The History of Anorexia Nervosa* (New York: Random House, 1988); and *From Fasting Saints to Anorexic Girls, the History of Self-starvation*. The quotes concerning the daughter of the English locksmith and Ann Moore are from *Fasting Girls*, pages 51–61. One original source is Hyder E. Rollins, "Notes on Some English Accounts of Miraculous Fasts," *Journal of American Folklore* 34 (1921).

The quote by Richard Foster is in his book *Celebration of Discipline, The Path to Spiritual Growth* (New York: HarperCollins Publishers, 1978), page 57.

The quotes by John Piper are from his book *A Hunger for God* (Wheaton, Illinois: Crossway Books, 1997), pages 14, 42, and 83. The quote by Mark Nysewander is from his book *The Fasting Key: How You Can Unlock Doors to Spiritual Blessing* (Ann Arbor: Vine Books, 2003), page 54.

Information on the renaissance of fasting can be found in Christine Gardner, "Hungry for God," *Christianity Today* 43, no. 4 (April 5, 1999), pages 32–38. This article explores the resurgence of fasting, details Jerry Falwell's fast, and lists the major fasts of the late 1990s. Another good discussion is by the editors of *Christianity Today* 43, no. 4 (April 5, 1999), pages 30–31, under the title "Not a Fast Fix." This essay is the source for the quote from John Piper, "Fasting is meant to awaken us to the hunger of the world. . . ." and the quote from Bob Pierce, founder of World Vision, "Break my heart with the things that break the heart of God." More information on The Call can be found at their website http://www.thecallrevolution.com. More information about World Vision can be found on their website http://www.worldvision.com.

The quote about the Korean churches is from *A Hunger for God*, page 103.

CHAPTER FIVE: THIRTY DAYS

The history of Henry Tanner and his fast comes from a number of sources. An especially good one is Hillel Schwartz, *Never Satisfied: A Cultural History of Diets, Fantasies, and Fat* (New York: Macmillan, 1986), pages 115–23. Schwartz also discusses other fasters and fasts of the late nineteenth and early twentieth century, such as Clare De Serval. Information about Tanner can be found as well in newspaper articles of that era, particularly the *New York Times* during the months of August and September of 1880, as well as Robert A. Gunn, *Forty Days Without Food, A Biography of Henry S. Tanner, M.D., Including a Complete and Accurate History of his Wonderful Fasts* (New York: Albert Metz and Company, 1890).

Information on A. Levanzin and his thirty-day fast can be found in Francis Gano Benedict, *A Study of Prolonged Fasting* (Washington, D.C.: Carnegie Institute of Washington, 1915). The description of Levanzin as a propagandist and his own refusal to ride a bicycle is on page 28. The description by scientists of Levanzin's personality and behavior is on page 213. Levanzin's journal entries are on page 27.

The material by Howard Marsh comes from his article "Individual and Sex Differences brought Out by Fasting," *Psychological Review* 23 (1916), pages 437–45.

The studies in 1910 and 1915 on therapeutic fasting and diabetes are in G. Guelpa, "Starvation and purgation in the relief of diabetes," *British Medical Journal* 2 (1910), pages 1050–51 and F. M. Allen, "Prolonged fasting in diabetes," *American Journal of Medical Science* 150 (1915), pages 480–85. The studies on fasting and epilepsy are W. G. Lennox, et al, "Studies in epilepsy," *Archives of Neurological Psychology* 20 (1928), pages 711–79; and "Ketone Bodies, Potential Therapeutic Uses."

The paper about the eleven fasting patients is Ernst J. Drenick, et al, "Prolonged Starvation as Treatment for Severe Obesity," *The Journal of the American Medical Association* (January 11, 1964), pages 140–45. The paper on the thirteen fasting patients is T. J. Thompson, et al, "Treatment of Obesity by Total Fasting for up to 249 Days," *The Lancet* (November 5, 1966), pages 992–96. The Scottish study is in "Features of a successful therapeutic fast of 382 days' duration."

A more complete bibliography of studies on the benefits of fasting can be found in books that promote fasting such as *Fasting and Eating for Health;* and Douglas Lisle and Alan Goldhamer, *The Pleasure Trap* (Summertown, Tennessee: Healthy Living Publications, 2003). More traditional articles in medical journals include one on the benefits of a seven-day fast in patients with bronchial asthma by Tovt-Korshyna'ka, et al, *Lik Sprava* 3–4 (April–June 2002), pages 79–81; on fasting therapy and chronic fatigue syndrome in Masuda A. Nakayama, et al, *Internal Medicine* 40, no. 11 (November 2001), pages 1158–61; on thirty-one reports of fasting studies on patients with rheumatoid arthritis in G. Muller, et al, *Scandinavian Journal of Rheumatology* 30, no. 1 (2001), pages 1–10; on the effects of fasts on blood thinning and clotting in M. Miertinen, et al, "Effect of fasting on fibrinolysis and blood coagulation," *American Journal of Cardiology* 10 (1962), pages 1142–48; on fasting and pancreatitis in S. Nvarro, et al, "Comparison of fasting, nasogastric suction and cimetidine in the treatment of acute pancreatitis," *Digestion* 30 (1984), pages 224–30; on fasting and detoxification in M. Imamura, et al, "A trial of fasting cure for PCB poisoned patients in Taiwan," *American Journal of Indian Medicine* 5 (1984), pages 147–53; and on fasting and ulcers in D. A. Johnston, et al, "The effects of fasting on 24-h gastric secretions of patients with duodenal ulcers resistant to ranitidine," *Alimentary Pharmacology Therapy* 3, no. 5 (1989), pages 471–79. The study on mice that model multiple sclerosis is in Vijay K. Kuchroo and Lindsay B. Nicholson, "Fast and Feel Good," *Nature* 422 (March 6, 2003), pages 27–28.

The history of therapeutic fasting can be found in a number of sources, including *From Fasting Saints to Anorexic Girls, the History of*

Self-starvation; and *Never Satisfied*. For information on how natural hygienic physicians view fasting, look at their various websites, as well as books like *Fasting and Eating for Health* and *The Pleasure Trap*.

Material on Alan Goldhamer and TrueNorth came from personal correspondence as well as *The Pleasure Trap*. For the study on hypertension, read Alan C. Goldhamer, et al, "Medically supervised Water-Only Fasting in the Treatment of Borderline Hypertension," *The Journal of Alternative and Complementary Medicine* 8, no. 5 (2002), pages 643–50; and Alan Goldhamer, et al, "Medically Supervised Water-fasting in the Treatment of Hypertension," *Journal of Manipulative and Physiological Therapeutics* 24, no. 5 (June 2001), pages 335–39.

A discussion of animal studies and calorie restriction can be found in "Starve Your Way to Health;" "Eat Less and Live Longer?"; and "Lean Times."

Articles on Biosphere II include Roy L. Walford, et al, "Physiologic Changes in Humans Subjected to Severe Calorie Restriction for Two Years in Biosphere 2: Health, Aging, and Toxicological Perspectives," *Toxicological Sciences*, Supplement 52 (1999), pages 61–65; Roy L. Walford, et al, "Caloric Restriction in Biosphere 2," *Journal of Gerontology* 57A, no. 6 (2002), pages B211–B224; and Roy L. Walford, et al, "The calorically restricted low-fat nutrient-dense diet in Biosphere 2 significantly lowers blood glucose, total leukocyte count, cholesterol, and blood pressure in humans," *Proceedings of the National Academy of Sciences* 89 (December 1992), pages 11533–37. Roy Walford was the science officer "aboard" Biosphere II and experienced this low-fat nutrient-dense diet firsthand. He went on to become a major proponent of calorie restriction, author of a number of books on the subject, and a man greatly revered by the members of the Calorie Restriction Society.

Two general reviews of how calorie restriction might benefit the body are "Calorie Restriction and aging: review of the literature and implications for studies in humans;" and "Caloric restriction and aging: an update."

The study concerning fasting mice has been widely reported. Look at "Intermittent fasting dissociates beneficial effects of dietary restriction on glucose metabolism and neuronal resistance to injury from calorie intake."

CHAPTER SIX: THE HUNGER STRIKE

A first-hand account of the suffragette movement is in E. Sylvia Pankhurst, *The Suffragette: The History of the Women's Militant Suffrage Movement, 1905–1910* (London, Gay and Hancock Limited, 1911). The quote concerning Mrs. Pankhurst's arrest comes from page 386. Another firsthand report is E. Sylvia Pankhurst, *The Suffrage Movement, an Intimate Account of Persons and Ideals* (London: Virago, 1931). The quotes concerning the first hunger strike are on page 307; the quote from the doctor in the newspaper is on page 318; the quotes on the "still life" and Sylvia's force feeding are on pages 442–44; the quote concerning the debate on hunger strikers in the House on Commons is on page 568, and the quote on the power of sacrifice is on page 588. Other historical sources are June Purvis, *Emmaline Pankhurst* (London: Routledge, 2002); George Klosko and Margaret Klosko, *The Struggle for Women's Rights, Theoretical and Historical Sources* (New Jersey: Prentice Hall, 1999); and Doris Stevens, *Jailed for Freedom: American Women Win the Vote* (Troutdale, Oregon: NewSage Press, 1995).

The quote from the Lord Mayor of Cork comes from Padraig O'Malley, *Biting at the Grave: the Irish Hunger Strikes and the Politics of Despair* (Boston: Beacon Press, 1990), page 26.

Material on the life of Mahatma Gandhi comes from Louis Fischer, *The Life of Mahatma Gandhi* (New York: Harper and Brothers, 1950). Gandhi's ideas about fasting for *Young India* was quoted in this book, page 233.

The quotes concerning Gandhi's fast against the young boys of the ashram in South Africa are from M. K. Gandhi, *The Story of My Experiments with Truth* (Washington, D.C.: Public Affairs Press, 1948), pages 418–20. In this autobiography, Gandhi also tells the story of his fast during the labor strike, pages 526–28. That material can also be found in Erik H. Erikson, *Gandhi's Truth* (New York: W. W. Norton and Company, 1969).

The quote on fasting to reform those who love me is from *The Life of Mahatma Gandhi*, page 156; the quote on friendship between Hindus and Moslems is on page 223; Louis Fisher's quote is on page 320; the quote from the letter to the Viceroy is on page 388; the quote in which he discusses his Delhi fast is on page 496; the quote in which he addresses the religious leaders is on page 499. His nine rules come from a 1924 article in *Young India*, also quoted in *The Life of Mahatma Gandhi*, page 234.

The material on the difference between obese and lean fasters is from "Hunger Disease"; and M. Elia, et al, "Differences in Fat, Carbohydrate, and Protein Metabolism between Lean and Obese Subjects Undergoing Total Starvation," *Obesity Research* 7, no. 6 (November 1999), pages 597–604.

A number of sources detail the story of the Irish Republican hunger strikers, including *Biting at the Grave* and David Beresford, *Ten Men Dead* (New York: Atlantic Monthly Press, 1987).

The reporter who made the statement concerning the validity of each death being dependent on the death that followed was Padraig O'Malley. *Biting at the Grave* is also the source of the statistic of at least 200 hunger strikes from 1972–82, page 25.

David Beresford tells the story of Paddy Quinn and his mother's intervention in *Ten Men Dead*, pages 266–70. The quote from the Quinn family statement comes from Padraig O'Malley, pages 121–22.

The quote from Bobby Sands is from the diary of Bobby Sands, March 1, 1981, which I accessed at http://larkspirit.com/hungerstrikes/diary.html.

The quotes from the manual on hunger strikes are from *Assistance for Hunger Strikes, a manual for physicians and other health personnel dealing with hunger strikers* (Netherlands: Johannes Wier Foundation for Health and Human Rights, 1995).

More information on current views concerning the ethics of hunger strikes can be found in George Annas, "Hunger Strikes," *British Medical Journal* 311, no. 7013 (October 28, 1995), pages 1114–15 and Lubomir Neoral, "Ethical and medico-legal problems concerning so-called hunger strikers," *Forensic Science International* 69 (1994), pages 327–28.

The quote on fasting is from *Gandhi's Truth,* page 417.

CHAPTER SEVEN: THE HUNGER DISEASE STUDIES

The quote by Viktor Frankl comes from his book *Man's Search for Meaning, an introduction to logotherapy* (New York: Simon and Schuster, 1962), pages 120–21.

The story of the Warsaw ghetto can be found in the well-researched book by Charles G. Roland, *Courage Under Siege: Starvation, Disease and Death in the Warsaw Ghetto* (New York: Oxford University Press, 1992). I also read Leonard Tushnet, *The Uses of Adversity* (New York: T. Yoseloff, 1966); Myron Winick, ed. and Martha Osnos, translator, *Hunger Disease: Studies by the Jewish Physicians in the Warsaw Ghetto* (New York: John Wiley and Sons, 1979); Raul Hilberg, et al, eds., *The Warsaw Diary of Adam Czerniakow* (New York: Stein and Day, 1979); Joseph Kermish, ed., *To Live With Honor and Die with Honor! Selected Documents from the Warsaw Ghetto Underground Archives,* (Jerusulem: Yad Vashem, 1986); Ulrich Keller, *The Warsaw Ghetto in Photographs* (New York: Dover Publications, 1984); and Abraham Lewin, *A Cup of Tears, A Diary of the Warsaw Ghetto* (Oxford: Basil Blackwell, 1988).

The quote by the German governor can be found in *The Uses of Adversity,* page 22. The quote about the children's songs comes from *To Live with Honor and Die with Honor! Selected Documents from the Warsaw Ghetto Underground Archives,* page 678. This section of the book includes some of the songs the children chanted and sang. The quote concerning the Berson and Bauman Hospital is in *Courage Under Siege,* page 180. The description of the boy in the hospital and the quote from the doctor pausing over the crib is from *To Live with Honor and Die with Honor! Selected Documents from the Warsaw Ghetto Underground Archives,* pages 401 and 404.

The information on the hunger disease studies is from *Hunger Disease*. Quoted material is from this translation.

The description of Dr. Anna Braude-Heller is in *Courage Under Siege,* page 94. The quote from the woman poisoning the babies is also from *Courage Under Siege,* page 180.

The fate of the scientists and researchers can be found in *The Uses of Adversity.*

CHAPTER EIGHT: THE MINNESOTA EXPERIMENT

The quote by Jack Drummond is in his foreword to volume one of Ancel Keys and Josef Brozak, et al, *The Biology of Human Starvation* (Minneapolis: University of Minnesota, 1950). The quote by the scientists concerning the nature of their work is from the introduction to this book. The quote from the proud volunteer is on page 903.

The activist who used the analogy to vegetarianism was Ammon Hennesey, quoted in the introduction to the television production *The Good War and Those Who Refused to Fight It,* produced and directed by Judith Ehrlich and Rick Tejada-Flores for the Independent Television Service. The quotes from the conscientious objectors complaining of their lack of significant work are from the introduction to Heather T. Frazer and John O'Sullivan, *We Have Just Begun To Not Fight, an oral history of conscientious objectors in Civilian Public Service during World War II* (New York: Twayne Publishers, 1996). This book also contains information about the medical experiments done with conscientious objectors during the war.

Jim Graham's quotes come from the video by B. Smith, *Minnesota Semi-Starvation Experiment,* Office of Instructional Services, Colorado State University, TV06684. This video also lists the advice given by Ancel Keys concerning the results of the Minnesota Experiment.

The material on the Minnesota Experiment is from *The Biology of Human Starvation.*

More information on Ancel Keys is in David Brown, "Keys of Nutrition," *The Washington Post* (October 22, 2002).

CHAPTER NINE: THE ANTHROPOLOGY OF HUNGER

Information on early anthropological research can be found in Audrey Richards, *Hunger and Work in a Savage Tribe: A Functional Study of Nu-*

trition among the Southern Bantu (Glencoe, Illinois: The Free Press, 1948); and in Allan R. Holmberg, *Nomads of the Long Bow* (New York: Natural History Press, 1969). The quotes from Holmberg's work can be found on pages 252 and 256.

Information on the Gurage can be found in Carole Counihan and Penny Van Esterik, eds., *Food and Culture, a reader*, (New York: Routledge Press, 1997), Chapter Ten; Dorothy Shack, "Nutritional Processes and Personality Development among the Gurage of Ethiopia," pages 118–23, and Chapter Eleven; and William Shack, "Hunger, Anxiety, and Ritual," pages 125–37.

Material on Kalauna is in Lenore Manderson, ed., *Shared Wealth and Society: Food, Culture, and Society in Oceania and Southeast Asia* (London: Cambridge University Press, 1986), Chapter Five; and Michael W. Young, "'The worst disease': the cultural definition of hunger in Kalauna," pages 113–26.

The story of the Ik comes from Colin Turnbull, *The Mountain People* (New York: Touchstone Books, 1972), with quotes from pages 12, 49, 123, and 265, as well as from Charles Laughlin, ed., *Extinction and Survival in Human Populations* (New York: Columbia University Press, 1978), Chapter Two; and Colin Turnbull, "Rethinking the Ik: A Functional Non-Social System," pages 48–75, with quotes from pages 62 and 72. I also read and enjoyed Roy Richard Grinker, *In the Arms of Africa: The Life of Colin Turnbull* (New York: St. Martin's Press, 2000). From this book, I used material that Grinker quotes from Turnbull's interview about the dysentery tablet, page 166, and from his interview with *The New Yorker*, page 173. The quote on Barth's criticism of Turnbull is from Fredrik Barth, "On Responsibility and Humanity: Calling a Colleague to Account," *Current Anthropology* 15, no. 1 (March 1974). The later critical report on Turnbull's work is Bernd Heine, "The Mountain People: Some Notes on the Ik of Northeastern Uganda," *Africa* 55, no. 1 (1985).

Robert Dirks's research is in his article "Social Responses during Severe Food Shortages and Famine," *Current Anthropology* 21, no. 1 (February 1980), pages 21–44.

Material on the famine in the Ukraine can be found in Miron Dolot, *Execution by Hunger, the Hidden Holocaust* (New York: W. W. Norton and Company, 1985). The famine in Leningrad is described in Harrison E. Salisbury, *The 900 Days, the Siege of Leningrad* (New York: Harper and Row Publishers, 1969). A short history of famines in China can be found in *Hunger in History*, Robin D. S. Yates, "War, Food Shortages and Relief Measures in Early China," pages 147–77. In the same book, also see Carl Riskin, "Food, Poverty, and Development Strategy in the People's Republic of China," pages 232–351.

Key Ray Chong is the author of *Cannibalism in China* (Wakefield, New Hampshire: Longwood Academic Press, 1990). His thesis is that the practice of cannibalism has a special place in China's history, playing many different roles and involving both "survival cannibalism" and "learned cannibalism." Chong believes that cannibalism was a recognized method of triumphing over or punishing one's enemy, and enemy soldiers were naturally considered as sources of food. Cannibalism could also be a gesture of self-sacrifice, as when daughters-in-law cut off parts of their thighs or buttocks to feed elderly parents. In addition, human flesh had medicinal and magical value and at times was considered a tasty dish. Chong's emphasis is not one found in traditional history books. The academic world seems to find his idea an interesting one that requires further research by more scholars. The material concerning the siege of 594 BC is on page 45 of *Cannibalism in China* and of the edict by Emperor Kao Tzu on page 64. This material is also in Jasper Becker, *Hungry Ghosts, Mao's Secret Famine* (New York: The Free Press, 1996). Another mention of widespread cannibalism in ancient Chinese history is in "War, Food Shortages, and Relief measures in Early China" and *Hunger in History*.

A contemporary account of cannibalism in China's recent famine is Zheng Yi, *Scarlet Memorial, Tales of Cannibalism in Modern China* (Boulder, Colorado: Westview Press, 1996). I also read Harry Wu, *Bitter Winds: A Memoir of My Years in China's Gulag* (New York: John Wiley and Sons, 1984), and Steven Mosher, *A Mother's Ordeal: One Woman's Fight Against China's One Child Policy* (New York: Harcourt and Brace and Company, 1993). A great resource and one of the few thorough accounts of the famine in China is *Hungry Ghosts, Mao's Secret Famine*. The quotes about cannibalism can be found on pages 118, 137–38, and 213. The quote about the mask of famine is from Zhang Xianliang, *Grass Soup* (Boston: David R. Godine, 1993), page 82. The final quote by Wei Jingsheng is from the *New York Times* (1980) also quoted in *Hungry Ghosts, Mao's Secret Famine*.

The quote from Nancy Scheper-Hughes praising Turnbull's work is in her book *Death Without Weeping: The Violence of Everyday Life in Brazil* (Berkeley: University of California Press, 1992), page 133. Her story and quotes come from this book, especially pages 138 and 174. I also read her account "The Madness of Hunger: Sickness, Delirium, and Human Needs," *Culture, Medicine and Psychiatry* 12 (1988), pages 429–58.

CHAPTER TEN: ANOREXIA NERVOSA

The quotes from *The Biology of Human Starvation* can be found in its chapter "Anorexia Nervosa and Pituitary Cachexia," pages 967–73.

Joan Jacobs Brumberg gives an overview of the history of anorexia nervosa in her book *Fasting Girls*, where she tells the story of Martha Taylor and John Reynold's "theory of fermentation." Another historical source is Jules Bemporad, "Self-starvation Through the Ages: Reflections on the Pre-history of Anorexia Nervosa" in *International Journal of Eating Disorders* 19, no. 3 (1996), pages 217–37. It is Brumberg who cautions, "Although Catherine of Siena and Karen Carpenter do have something in common—the use of food as a symbolic language—it is as inappropriate to call the former an anorectic as it is to cast the latter as a saint. To describe pre-modern women such as Catherine as anorexic is to flatten differences in female experience across time. . . ."

The quote from Sigmund Freud is from his book *The Origin and Development of Psychoanalysis* (New York: Basic Books, 1889/1954), page 201.

The information from the National Association of Anorexia and Associated Disorders can be found on their website http://www.amad. org. In Pamela Hardin, "Shape-shifting discourses of anorexia nervosa:

reconstituting psychopathology," *Nursing Inquiry* 10, no. 4 (2003), pages 209–17 is a discussion of media stories and websites promoting anorexia nervosa. The rise of eating disorders in middle age is in Ginia Bellafante, "When Midlife Seems Just an Empty Plate," the *New York Times*, Section 9 (March 9, 2003). The article cited a study from *International Journal of Eating Disorders* in which patients ages 40–49 account for 9 percent of admissions to a Cornell University hospital. In 1985, Gerald F. M. Russell wrote about "The Changing Nature of Anorexia Nervosa" in *Journal of Psychiatric Review* 19, no. 2/3 (1985), pages 101–9. The increases he discussed were not limited to the United States; Russell noted "a five-fold increase in Malmo, Sweden between the 1930s and the 1950s" and, in 1985, "even greater increases have been reported in north-east Scotland, with a rise in annual incidence from 1.6 to 4.1 per 1000." A more recent discussion is in Hans Hoek, et al, "Review of the Prevalence and Incidence of Eating Disorders," *International Journal of Eating Disorders* 34, no. 4 (2003), pages 384–97. After reviewing the literature, this article cites a lower incidence of anorexia nervosa than NAAAD (an average of .3 for young females) and sees a rise in the disease from the 1950s into the 1970s followed by a stabilization.

There are various death rates given for anorexia nervosa. A good discussion of this range and of other medical concerns, including heart problems and osteoporosis, is in Philip Mehler, et al, "Anorexia Nervosa Medical Issues," *Journal of Women's Health* 12, no. 4 (2003), pages 331–39. Also, see S. Zipfel, et al, "Long-term prognosis in anorexia nervosa: lessons from a 21-year follow-up study," *The Lancet* 355 (2000), pages 721–22.

The article "The Hunger Artists" in *U.S. News and World Reports*, June 10, 2002, pages 45–50, gives a good popular update on the biology and genetics of anorexia nervosa. Dr. Hans Hoek's quote and work is described in the BBC program "Fat Files—Living on Air," which can be found at http://diglander.libero.it/rrosalia/tisorse/bbc.html. Elke Elkart's research covers a range of issues in anorexia nervosa. I depended on personal correspondence and the audiotape of Elkart's paper "Long-term Effects of Semi-starvation on Eating Patterns: Follow-up to the Keys Study, Implications for Practitioners" delivered at a conference of the American Dietetic Association on April 5–7, 2002, in Orlando, Florida. Another discussion of the Minnesota Experiment in relation to anorexia nervosa is in Daniel Garner and P. E. Garfinkel, *D.M.*, *Handbook for Treatment of Eating Disorders* (New York: Guilford Press, 1997). The study on fat can be found in Steven Grinspoon, et al, "Changes in regional fat redistribution and the effects of estrogen during spontaneous weight gain in women with anorexia nervosa" in *American Journal of Clinical Nutrition* 73 (2001), pages 865–69.

Jennifer Shute's quotes are from her novel *Life Size* (Boston: Houghton-Mifflin Company, 1992). Caroline Knapp's quotes are from *Appetites: Why Women Want* (New York: Counterpoint, 2003). Other accounts of eating disorders, which include binging and overeating are Cherry Boone O'Neil, *Starving for Attention* (New York: Continuum Press, 1982); Margaret Bullit-Jonas, *Holy Hunger: A Memoir of Desire* (New York: Alfred Knopf, 1999); and Steven Levenkron, *Anatomy of Anorexia* (New York: W. W. Norton and Company, 2000).

The basic theory of anorexia nervosa as an evolutionary adaptation is in Shan Guisinger, "Adapted to Flee: Adding an Evolutionary Perspective on Anorexia Nervosa," *Psychological Review* 110, no. 4 (2002), pages 745–61. Two IRA prisoners, Marian and Dolores Price, began hunger strikes while in prison and later developed anorexia nervosa. More information can be found in Miriam O'Kane Mara, "A Famine of Preference: Images of Anorexia in Contemporary Irish Literature," Dissertation (Albuquerque: University of New Mexico, August 2003).

Susan Bordo's quote is from her essay "Anorexia Nervosa: Psychopathology as the crystallization of Culture," *Philosophical Forum* 17, no. 2 (Winter 1985). Michell Mary Lelwica's quote from an anorectic is in her book *Starving for Salvation* (New York: Oxford University Press, 1999), page 106. The quote by Rachel Fentem about anorexia being her best friend is in the BBC program "Fat Files—Living on Air."

CHAPTER ELEVEN: HUNGRY CHILDREN

The material on the Dutch Hunger Winter comes from many sources, including the seminal study Zena Stein, et al, *Famine and Human Development: The Dutch Hunger Winter of 1944–45* (New York: Oxford University Press, 1975). This book is the source of the information about starvation hospitals, page 46, as well as the statistics on the effect of prenatal famine based on hospital records of that time and the records kept by the Dutch military, including the material on mental disease and development. The study from the 1970s on obesity and the Dutch Hunger Winter is in Gian-Paolo Ravelli, et al, "Obesity in Young Men After Famine Exposure in Utero and Early Infancy," *The New England Journal of Medicine* 295, no. 7 (August 12, 1976), pages 349–53. The study of 700 subjects in their fifties is in Gian-Paulo Ravelli, et al, "Obesity at the age of 50 years in men and women exposed to famine prenatally," *American Journal of Clinical Nutrition* 70 (1999), pages 811–16. The study on sex differences and neurodevelopmental disorders is in Ezra Susser, Hans Hoek, et al, "Neurodevelopmental Disorders after Prenatal Famine," *American Journal of Epidemiology* 147, no. 3 (1998), pages 213–16. The study concerning cholesterol levels is in Tess Rosenboom, et al, "Plasma lipid profiles in adults after prenatal exposure to the Dutch famine," *American Journal of Clinical Nutrition* 72 (2000), pages 1101–06. Studies that connect prenatal famine to mental diseases are Alan S. Brown, Hans Hoek, et al, "Prenatal Famine and the Spectrum of Psychosis," *Psychiatric Annals* 29, no. 3 (March 1999), pages 145–50; Hulshoff, Hilleke, et al, "Prenatal exposure to famine and brain morphology in schizophrenia," *American Journal of Psychiatry* 157, no. 7 (July 2000), pages 1170–72; and Alan S. Brown, Hans Hoek, et al, "Further Evidence of Relation Between Prenatal Famine and Major Affective Disorder," *American Journal of Psychiatry* 157, no. 2 (February 2000), pages 190–95.

The quote from Charles Dickens is in Kenneth F. Kiple and Kiremhild Conee Ornelas, *The Cambridge World History of Food* (Cambridge: Cambridge University Press, 2000), page 979. This book is a good overview of the causes of child malnutrition and the history of our understanding of this disease; it is also the source for the statistic on child deaths in New York in 1915.

Original material about kwashiorkor is from Cicely Williams, et al, "Kwashiorkor, a nutritional disease of children associated with a maize diet," *The Lancet* 229 (November 16, 1935), pages 912–13. My description of kwashiorkor also comes from personal correspondence with Michael Golden.

The quote from the 1956 study on the psychology of kwashiorkor is in M. Geber and R. F. A. Dean, "The psychological changes accompanying kwashiorkor," *Courier* 6, no. 1 (1956).

One overview of child malnutrition and the history of research in this field can be found in Zulfiqar Ahmed Bhutta, *Contemporary Issues in Childhood Diarrhea and Malnutrition* (New York: Oxford University Press, 2000); and J. C. Waterlow, "Current Concepts of the Pathogenesis of Protein-Energy Malnutrition (PEM) in Childhood," pages 26–37. For an understanding of the physiology, I also depended on David Warrell, et al, *Oxford Textbook of Medicine*, 4th ed. (Oxford: Oxford University Press, 2003); Alan Jackson, "Severe malnutrition," pages 1054–61

The study concerning the Indonesian preschoolers is in A. Sommer, et al, "Impact of Vitamin A Supplementation on Childhood Mortality," *The Lancet* (1986), pages 1169–73.

Michael Golden's contributions to the understanding of child malnutrition are many. I relied on Michael Golden, "Oedmatous Malnutrition," *British Medical Bulletin* 54, no. 2 (1998), pages 433–44; Michael Golden, "The Development of the Concept of Malnutrition," *American Society for Nutritional Sciences*, Supplement 2002; Michael Golden and D. Ramdath, "Free radicals in the pathogenesis of kwashiorkor," *Proceedings of the Nutrition Society* 46 (1987), pages 53–68; and Michael Golden, "Trace Elements in Human Nutrition," *Human Nutrition: Clinical Nutrition* (1982), pages 185–202. Dr. Golden and I also corresponded personally. His quote concerning oxidation and "going rancid" is from an interview with the U.N. Office for the Coordination of

Humanitarian Affairs on Monday, 14 June 2004, which can be found at http://www.irinnews.org.

The number of eleven children dying every minute from hunger-related causes and the percentage of malnourished children in low-income countries come from the nonprofit organization Concern Worldwide; more information can be found on their website http://www.concernworldwide. org. They estimate that 60 percent of deaths of children under five years of age are associated with undernutrition—or 3.7 million deaths annually. The numbers of stunted and malnourished children in the world come from the World Health Organization. See http://www.who.int/en, as well as other organizations dealing with world hunger and malnutrition.

The story of the 1984 BBC film is in Susan Moeller, *Compassion Fatigue: How the Media Sells Disease, Famine, War, and Death* (New York: Routledge Publishers, 1999), pages 111–17. The quote on children as the "famine icon" is on page 99. Moeller's quotes concerning Kevin Carter are on pages 146–49, including the quote to his friend, originally from articles in *The Sunday Mail* and *The Village Voice*. This information on the 1984 BBC film is in other sources as well, including Jenny Edkins, *Whose Hunger?: Concepts of Famine, Practices of Aid* (Minneapolis: University of Minnesota Press, 2000). Edkins's book is an absorbing exploration of how famines have been seen and understood in the twentieth century. The quote on Somalia concerning the "blind, fly-ridden girl" is also in *Compassion Fatigue* and comes originally from an article by Jack Kelly, *USA Today* (September 9, 1992).

More information on malnutrition and cognition is in David Levitsky and Barbara Strupp, "Malnutrition and the Brain: Changing Concepts, Changing Concerns," *Journal of Nutrition* 125, no. 8 (August 1995), pages 2212–20. I also read the "Statement on the Link Between Nutrition and Cognitive Development in Children," Center on Hunger and Poverty (1998), which can be found on their website http://www.centeronhunger.org/cognitive.html; and Michelle Mendez, et al, "Severity and Timing of Stunting in the First Two Years of Life Affect Performance on Cognitive Tests in Late Childhood," *American Society for Nutritional Sciences* (1999), pages 1555–62.

Information on the Guatemalan studies can be found in Ernesto Pollitt, et al, "Nutrition in Early Life and the Fulfillment of Intellectual Potential," *American Institute of Nutrition* Supplement (1995), pages 1111–18; and in J. Larry Brown and Ernesto Pillitt, "Malnutrition, Poverty, and Intellectual Development," *Scientific American* (February 1996), pages 38–43. The study on Jamaican children and play therapy is in S. M. Grantham-McGregor, et al, "Nutritional Supplementation, Psychosocial Stimulation, and Mental Development of Stunted Children: The Jamaican Study," *The Lancet* 338 (July 1991), pages 1–5 and S. M. Grantham-McGregor, "Effect of early childhood supplementation with and without stimulation on later development in stunted Jamaican children," *The American Journal of Clinical Nutrition* 66, no. 2 (August 1997), pages 247–53.

The studies in Barbados that show that children with earlier severe malnutrition have a high rate of attention deficit disorder and a significant drop in IQ compared to control groups include J. R. Galler, "A follow-up study on the influence of early malnutrition on development: behavior at home and at school," *Journal of American Academy of Child and Adolescent Psychiatry* 28, no. 2 (March 1989), pages 254–61; and J. R. Galler, et al, "The influence of early malnutrition on subsequent behavioral development," *Pediatric Research* 18, no. 4 (April 1984), pages 309–13.

Studies on the effect of the home environment on buffering malnutrition are in David Barrett and Deborah Frank, *The Effects of Undernutrition on Children's Behavior* (New York: Gordon and Breach Science Publishers, 1987).

The study on children in Worcester, Massachusetts, is in Linda Weinreb, et al, "Hunger: Its Impact on Children's Health and Mental Health," *Pediatrics* 110, no. 4 (October 2002), pages 41–44.

Information on the care of malnourished children comes from "Management of the Child with a Serious Infection or Severe Malnutrition," World Health Organization (2000).

In personal correspondence and in articles and drafts of articles, Dr. Golden urges that the WHO guidelines be further refined. He and his colleagues have worked on these refinements in the field and have written up their results in articles like F. Buhendwa, et al, "Death during treatment for severe malnutrition: effect of medication of the standard protocols in Kinshea," (unpublished). The new instructions would emphasize, strongly, that any severely malnourished child should be given sugar water rather than any solution with salt and that blood transfusions should be limited. Golden wants to tinker with a number of other strategies, such as advice about breastfeeding, which formulas to use, and why not to give IVs. He would also refine the procedure for specific situations, like the hot deserts of Sudan. His own research shows that with updated protocols the death rate can drop below current WHO expectations.

CHAPTER TWELVE: PROTOCOLS OF FAMINE

Information on Steve's work in Baidoa comes from personal communication, as well as Steve Collins, "The limits of human adaptation to starvation," *Nature Medicine* 1, no. 8 (August 1995), pages 810–15 and Steve Collins, Mark Myatt, and Barbara Golden, "Dietary treatment of severe malnutrition in adults," *American Journal of Clinical Nutrition* 68 (1998), pages 193–99.

Material on treating adults is in Steve Collins, "The need to treat adults during famine relief," *JAMA* (August 1993) and Steve Collins and Peter Salama, "An Ongoing Omission: Adolescent and Adult Malnutrition in Famine Situations," *Emergency Nutrition Network* (1998).

Steve's story of his experience in Liberia can be found in Steve Collins, "The Risks of Wet Feeding Programmes," an article accessed on http://www.validinternational.org. Information on the relationship of disease and hunger comes from many sources, including Helen Young and Susanne Jaspar, "Nutrition, Disease, and Death in Times of Famine," *Disasters* 19, no. 2 (1995), pages 94–109; *Oxford Textbook of Medicine;* "Severe malnutrition;" and Joel Mokyr, "Famine Disease and Famine Mortality: Lessons from Ireland, 1845–1850, Thesis (Chicago: Northwestern University, 1999).

Steve's discussion of three clinical signs as predictors in Baidoa is in Steve Collins and Mark Myatt, "Short-term Prognosis in Severe Adult and Adolescent Malnutrition During Famine," *JAMA* 264, no. 4 (August 2, 2000), pages 621–26. For his "Chances model," see Steve Collins, Arabella Duffield, and Mark Myatt, "Assessment of Nutritional Status in Emergency-affected Populations," *RNIS*, Supplement (July 2000).

The discussion of the famine in the Sudan and the material concerning prioritization of resources is in Andre Griekspoor and Steve Collins, "Raising standards in emergency relief: how useful are Sphere minimum standards for humanitarian assistance?" *British Medical Journal* 323 (September 29, 2001), pages 740–42.

A description of outpatient care in Ethiopia in 2000 is in Kate Sadler and Steve Collins, "Outpatient care for severely malnourished children in emergency relief programmes: a retrospective cohort study," *The Lancet* 360 (December 7, 2002), pages 1824–30 and in Steve Collins, "Changing the way we address severe malnutrition during famine," *The Lancet*. 358 (August 11, 2001), pages 498–501.

A comprehensive discussion of CTC can be found in Steve Collins, "Community-Based Therapeutic Care for acute malnutrition" (Valid International, 2004), which can be found on the website http://www.validinternational.org. Online access to many of the articles authored by Steve Collins, as well as details on all of Valid International's projects, can also be found on this website.

I read a number of general books on famine, including Patrick Webb and Joachim von Braun, *Famine and Food Security* (New York: John Wiley and Sons, 1994); *Whose Hunger?*; and Barnett Rubon, ed., *The Geopolitics of Hunger, 2000–2201, Hunger and Power* (Boulder, Colorado: Lynne Rienner Publishers, 2001).

Interestingly, after her experiences with the suffragettes, Sylvia Pankhurst went on to travel and ultimately devote the rest of her life to the people of Ethiopia. In Alulu Pankhurst, *Resettlement and Famine in Ethiopia, the villagers' experience* (Manchester, New York: Manchester University Press, 1992), Sylvia's granddaughter Alulu Pankhurst writes of famine as "a modern myth of apocalyptic magnitude. The vision of living skeletons shown on television screens propagated a message of passive resignation and silent despair." And yet, "Aid workers in shelters recall that for every living corpse the cameraman honed in on there were a hundred dignified undernourished people awaiting their fate. Likewise, for every person who decided to walk to the shelters, there were hundreds who sought different ways to eke out a living, gathering wild plants, rationing reserve and selling assets, migrating in search of wage-labor, taking part in food-for-work projects."

CHAPTER THIRTEEN: AN END TO HUNGER

Some of my experiences in Guatemala were originally published in my essay "Guatemala" in the literary magazine *Puerto del Sol*.

For more information on the Millennium Goals and on the Hunger Task Force, see the interim report of the Millennium Project Hunger Task Force, "Halving Hunger by 2015: A Framework for Action," at their website http://www.unmillenniumproject.org, as well as their executive summary by Sara Scherr, et al, "Background Paper of the Millennium Task Force on Hunger," April 18, 2003. Another website that focuses on the Hunger Task Force and contains these two reports is http://www. earthinstitute.columbia.edu. I also read Tom Arnold, "Ethics, Politics, and Policies in World Hunger," (unpublished paper) and Tom Arnold, "Catalysts for change," *Global Agenda 2004*, pages 87–88. More information about Concern Worldwide can be found on their website http://www.concern.net.

The blueprint to ending hunger in America can be found in "A Blueprint to End Hunger" (National Anti-Hunger Organizations, June 3, 2004), which can be downloaded from http://www.hungercenter.org.

CHAPTER FOURTEEN: THE TOP OF THE MOUNTAIN

There are many sources for the story of Saint Patrick's life. I used J. M. Holmes, *The Real Saint Patrick* (Ballyclare: Irish Hill Publications, 2002), which includes translations by Ludwig Bieler of Saint Patrick's "Confession" and "Letter to Coroticus." Most historians judge these two Latin works to be genuine, written by Patrick in the fifth century. For some of the legends surrounding Saint Patrick, I also read George Otto

Simms, *Saint Patrick: Ireland's Patron Saint* (Dublin: O'Brien Press, 2004). I recommend Thomas Cahill, *How the Irish Saved Civilization* (New York: Doubleday, 1995) for a longer, lively discussion of Patrick and his adventures in history.

In fact, Ireland has no snakes today and probably never did, being both cold and an island.

Material about fasting in early Irish law can be found in Fergus Kelly, *A Guide to Early Irish Law*, (Dublin: Dublin Institute for Academic Studies: Early Irish Law Series, 1988) and in D. A. Binchy, "Irish History and Irish Law," *Studia Hibernica*, no. 15 (1975). Binchy also describes the legend in which Saint Patrick fasts against God and believes this to be a confused mergence of the "Christian *aine*, an ascetic practice, and the pre-Christian *troscad*, a method of enforcing claims against one's superiors." He notes the parallel between Irish and Indian practices and wonders if the "legal remedies represented a peripheral survival of an archaic practice once common to all the people who spoke an Indo-European language."

Some of the information on pilgrimages comes from *Walking in Ireland* (London: Lonely Planet, 1999), as does the quote about the summer holiday season.

The history of Ireland comes from a number of general sources. For material about the Great Famine and earlier famines, I relied on the classic Cecil Woodham-Smith, *The Great Hunger, Ireland 1845–1849* (London: Penguin Books, 1962); Peter Gray, *The Irish Famine* (London: Thames and Hudson, 1995); and Cathal Poirteir, *The Great Irish Famine* (Ireland: Merceir Press, 1995).

An important source for material on earlier famines, the role of the potato in the Irish diet, and comparisons of Irish famines with those in England and Europe was L. A. Clarkson and E. Margaret Crawford, *Feast and Famine: Food and Nutrition in Ireland 1500–1920* (London: Oxford Press, 2001).

The quote from the visitor to Galway is from Woodham-Smith's *The Great Hunger*, page 92. The quote on the blight is also from *The Great Hunger*, page 91. Descriptions of diseases during the famine are in the above mentioned books. The quote about relief funds buying arms is in Woodham-Smith's *The Great Hunger*, page 105. I also used "Famine Disease and Famine Mortality: Lessons from Ireland, 1845–50."

An overview of Great Hunger memorials in the United States is in Jane Holtz Kay, "Hunger for Memorials," *Landscape Architecture* (March 2003).

Gabriel Byrne's quote is from his essay "Famine Walk" in Tom Hayden, *Irish Hunger* (Boulder: Robert Rinehart Publishers, 1997). The novel by Nuala O'Faolain is *My Dream of You* (New York: Riverhead Books, 2001). The quote by Mary Robinson comes from her book *A Voice for Somalia* (Dublin: O'Brien Press, 1992).

ACKNOWLEDGMENTS

Many people helped me with this book. First, of course, are those scientists and humanitarian aid workers who gave me their time in personal interviews and conversations by email. Angelo Del Parigi was a gracious host during my visit to his lab in Phoenix; I hope this country remains a good host to him as well. Elizabeth Pearce at the Roadrunner Food Bank in Albuquerque took me on a tour of her world. Alan Goldhamer at TrueNorth Health Center was always gracious. Elke Eckert kindly looked over the material concerning her research. Michael Golden was generous with his time and comments. Meeting up in Dublin with Steve Collins of Valid International was pure serendipity; I am very grateful for his help. Tom Arnold, executive director of Concern Worldwide, very hospitably invited me into his home and office.

A number of friends also read over parts of this book. Patty Reed showed me what was missing in the first chapter. Dr. Fred Fox, who took my anxious call when I was three days a-fasting, patiently explained the mechanics of blood pressure. Dr. Bill Neely and Cindy Chvala are good readers, as well as good cooks. Dr. Moyra Smith helped me enormously with her eye for medical detail and her own interest and passion for the subject of hunger and humanitarian assistance. Kate Haake was always there with moral support. My husband, Peter Russell, read the entire rough draft and offered his comments and cheer. My daughter Maria Russell served as a research assistant and a wonderful companion on our trip to Ireland. Amanda Cook at Perseus Books first helped champion this book. Megan Hustad at Basic Books followed through on the project with insightful comments and smart editing.

I would also like to thank The Rockefeller Foundation in New York for granting me a four-week fellowship at their study and convention center in Bellagio, Italy. Certainly it seemed ironic at times to be writing about hunger while surrounded by such luxury and beauty. But hunger is ironic, and I quickly adjusted. During these weeks, Linda and Jim McMichaels were especially good friends and dinner companions.

Part of Chapter One, on pregnancy and famine, appeared earlier in an essay "Feast and Famine" in *The Sun: A Magazine of Ideas*. A section of Chapter Thirteen was first told in "Guatemala" in the literary magazine *Puerto del Sol: A Journal of Literature and Fine Art*.

As always, I need to thank the Interlibrary Loan Department of Miller Library at Western New Mexico University. How else could I write books? The many authors to whom I am greatly indebted are all detailed in the closing selected bibliography. Finally, I'd like to acknowledge the administration at Western New Mexico University and the faculty, staff, and students at the MFA program at Antioch University in Los Angeles for their general enthusiasm and support.